MAKE CHANGE THAT LASTS

9 Simple Ways to Break Free from the Habits That Hold You Back

DR. RANGAN CHATTERJEE

Photography by Rich Gilligan

BenBella Books, Inc.
Dallas, TX

BenBella

BenBella Books, Inc.
8080 N. Central Expressway
Suite 1700
Dallas, TX 75206
benbellabooks.com
Send feedback to feedback@benbellabooks.com

BenBella is a federally registered trademark.

Printed in the United States of America
10 9 8 7 6 5 4 3 2 1

Library of Congress Cataloging-in-Publication Data is available upon request.
ISBN 9781637747261 (print)
ISBN 9781637745991 (ebook)

Cover design by Sarah Avinger
Cover photo by Rich Gilligan

**Special discounts for bulk sales are available.
Please contact bulkorders@benbellabooks.com.**

To all who seek meaningful change that lasts

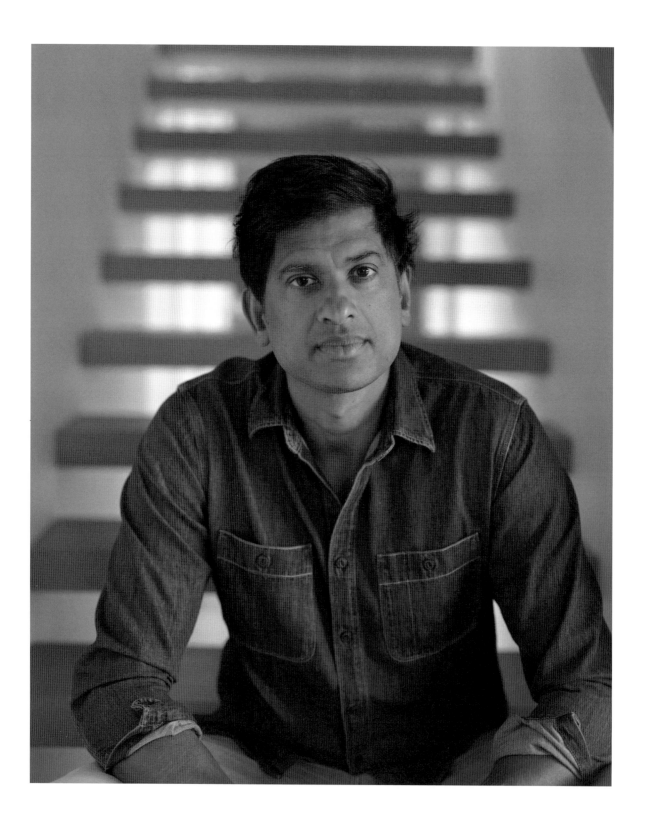

CONTENTS

INTRO-
DUCTION

MAKE CHANGE THAT LASTS

As soon as I answered the call, I could tell my old friend Helen was in a bad way. Helen had been a GP for sixteen years and was one of the most resilient, positive people I knew. Despite the grueling demands made on her in her inner-city practice, I'd never once heard her complain. She was a brilliant doctor who cared deeply about people. I felt lucky to know her. But on the phone that morning, I was surprised to hear her voice break as she asked if she could discuss something with me, face to face. Something was definitely wrong.

When we met for coffee that weekend, Helen explained that she'd had a run-in with a patient that had left her deeply upset. This patient was pre-diabetic, and she was talking to him about modifying his diet. There weren't many GPs who were more knowledgeable than Helen about the damage that too many ultra-processed and sugary foods can do to the body. She was a true expert in the field, always up to date with the latest peer-reviewed studies, many of which she would email me, alongside her own informed and fascinating commentary. She was carefully explaining to this patient how excess sugar can increase his levels of inflammation, when he said to her, "Why should I listen to you? You're fatter than I am."

I was shocked to hear this and felt terrible for Helen. But as Helen herself pointed out to me, her patient was right. "God, it was so humiliating," she told me. "I just didn't know what to say." She shook her head and laughed sadly. "I'm lecturing him about the harmful effects of sugar, when I've got a bag of Cadbury's giant buttons sitting right there in my desk drawer."

Helen had been trying to control her chocolate habit for years. The reason she had become so well versed in the science of unhealthy eating, she told me, was because

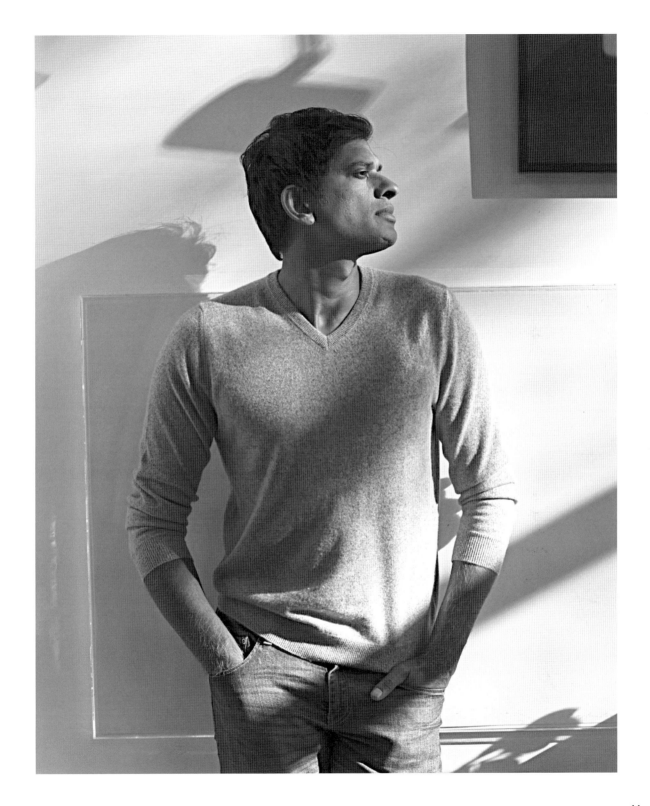

she had been trying to educate herself into having a better diet. "It clearly hasn't worked," she sighed. "I know everything there is to know, pretty much. I know sugar is harming my health and now, apparently, it's harming my ability to help my patients. But I still can't stop. There's always some excuse I manage to come up with to treat myself, you know? I don't know what to do."

I immediately thought of some of my own patients, who seemed to already know everything I could tell them about health and yet, despite being desperate for change, somehow couldn't turn their knowledge into action. I also thought about the listeners of my podcast, *Feel Better, Live More*, and the readers of my books. So many times I'd spoken to people who were enthusiastic and committed to learning about health and made absolutely sure they were up to date on the latest ideas and findings, but still struggled massively to achieve the change they were so desperate for. They might be eating too much sugar, like Helen, or ultra-processed foods, or drinking too much caffeine or alcohol. They might be struggling to manage their stress or sleeping poorly. They might be failing to move their body enough. I could think of so many people who knew perfectly well what they should be doing, and why they should be doing it, but were still unable to make the final brave leap to successful change. They had all found what Helen had also discovered: that – sometimes – knowledge is not enough.

How could I help these people? What was going on with them? What, exactly, was the short-circuit that needed fixing?

"Knowledge is not enough."

INSIGHT VERSUS OUTSIGHT

This book is the result of years of deep thinking about how to help anyone who finds themself in Helen's position. It will teach you how to achieve the life you want, not by looking outside to the wider world for the latest facts, findings and health trends, but by looking inside. Because inside is where so many of our problems begin.

Unhealthy habits are always seen as a cause of ill-health. Get rid of the habit, then you'll improve your health. This sounds so easy, but we all know that it's anything but. I believe it's hard because we've got the concept of unhealthy habits all wrong. Instead of being a cause of problems that need to be somehow eradicated, I see unhealthy habits as a symptom of other upstream problems – problems that are, very often, completely invisible to us.

An individual's overconsumption of sugar, for example, may be their way of dealing with a toxic work environment. Someone else's excess alcohol consumption may be their way of dealing with unresolved issues in their intimate relationships. In order to get rid of the downstream symptom, we have to first identify its upstream cause. This means developing our powers of insight.

I think of it as being the difference between a thermostat and a thermometer. Helen was a brilliantly effective thermometer. She knew everything there was to know about the harm caused by the overconsumption of sugar. Just like a thermometer, she had the power of "outsight" – the ability to look out into the world and read its information. She could use her excellent outsight to make a judgement on how well, or how badly, she was doing. But that's all she could do. She didn't have the power to actually change anything. For that, she'd have to become a thermostat. A thermostat has outsight but also insight – it has the knowledge and the power that enables it to change what it needs to change to achieve its ideal temperature.

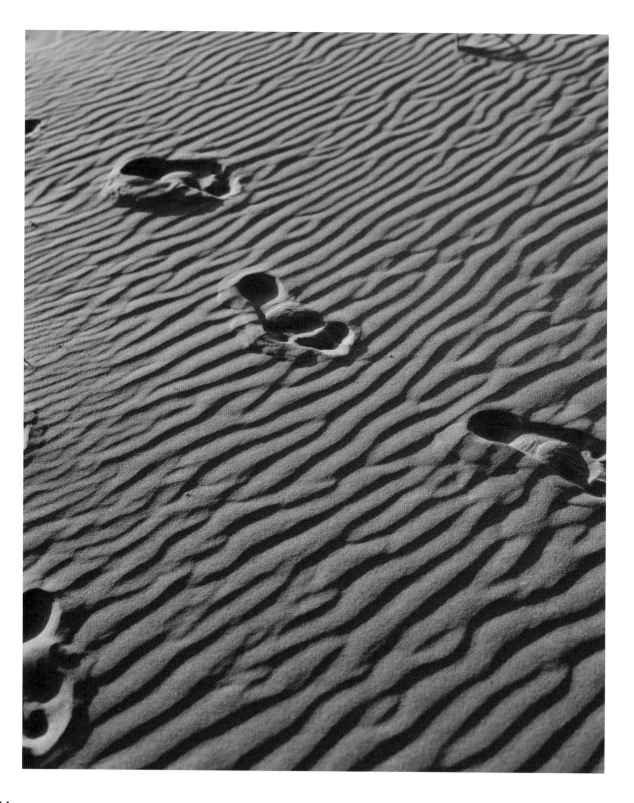

MEET YOUR INVISIBLE RELIANCES

By learning the art and practice of looking inside ourselves, we can discover the hidden causes of our unwanted behaviors. Almost without exception, the stubborn habits that damage our health and wellbeing are an escape from inner discomfort. As we go through our days, we inevitably encounter many situations that have the potential to generate emotional stress and internal tension. This stress and tension has to be neutralized somehow. Most of us do it mindlessly, by relying on unhealthy yet soothing habits, whether it's doomscrolling on our phones, drinking alcohol or gorging on sugar, carbs or highly processed foods. By becoming conscious of the situations that trigger these responses, we can respond to them intentionally and make changes that actually last.

I'd like you to start thinking about your emotional triggers as "reliances." Without really being aware of it, we all have different things we rely on, in order to feel calm and happy. Why not take a moment to make a rough list of all the things, large and small, that you're reliant upon to feel good? What's on your list? Do you need your partner to have woken up in a good mood? Your children to have put their shoes away and to not be arguing? For your smartphone to be always at hand? For there to be no terrible news in the morning headlines? For there to be no opinions you don't agree with on social media? For there to be no heavy traffic or bad drivers on your way to the school, office or station? For there to be someone you admire leading the country? For there to be no racism, homophobia or misogyny in the world? Do you need to be pleased with the reflection you see in the mirror? For there to be no new signs of increased weight or aging? Do you need your boss to be always kind, generous and complimentary towards you? Do you need lines in coffee shops and supermarkets never to be too long and for checkout staff to always be polite and efficient? Do you need the weather to be neither too hot nor too cold and for the wind to not be blowing too hard?

If you're anything like me, you'll find this simple thought experiment a little jarring. When I first did this exercise around five years ago or so, it felt like I could go on listing things forever. I realized that waking up to rain would often put my mood off and traffic on the way to work would leave me feeling frustrated – which, if you really think about it, is crazy. How could I expect to live my life to the fullest when I was being tied down by all these invisible needs and expectations, all of which were completely outside my control?

MINIMAL RELIANCE

Every individual reliance we have ties us to the ground and prevents us from thriving. When we're over-reliant, we're like the hero of the famous book *Gulliver's Travels*, bound to the ground by an army of tiny Lilliputians who are intent on keeping us prisoner. Every invisible reliance is a separate point of risk. Yes, we're able to feel somewhat good when some of them are met. On the rare occasions when most of them are met we can even feel extremely good. But the cost of all that reliance is vulnerability. We're giving our power and agency away and putting our wellbeing in the hands of people and forces that we can't control.

This is a huge problem, especially in an era in which many of us are already feeling out of control. Our lives are increasingly complex and demanding. It wasn't that long ago that one parent could afford to look after their children full-time, while the other went to a job that was often "nine to five." The working partner would be home by six and they'd be able to enjoy evenings and weekends together as a family, with the shops shut on Sundays. There are many reasons to see this kind of life as antiquated and contrary to modern values, and I understand them fully. My point is that this was a simpler, less stressful existence, one that was completely normal until relatively recently. Today's family has to endure far more pressure if, as is usual, both parents work. And even if you don't have children, there is still a cultural pressure to overwork and balance in life feels hard to achieve. On top of this we have smartphones and constant access to social media, which has surely played a huge part in the surge in mental health problems that we now see. Then there are the various crises we have lurched from over the last few years, one after the other – from the global financial crisis all the way up to the cost-of-living crisis, with the COVID pandemic happening in between. With all of this going on, it's almost impossible for every single one of our reliances to be met; as a consequence, we feel our lives are out of control.

When we feel out of control, we feel stressed and anxious. When we feel stressed and anxious, we often seek short-term release from discomfort in the form of an unhealthy habit. This is why I believe it makes sense to radically reduce our reliance on a world that is –and always will be – almost entirely uncontrollable. If you follow the advice in these pages, you will achieve a state of freedom and inner power that I call "Minimal Reliance."

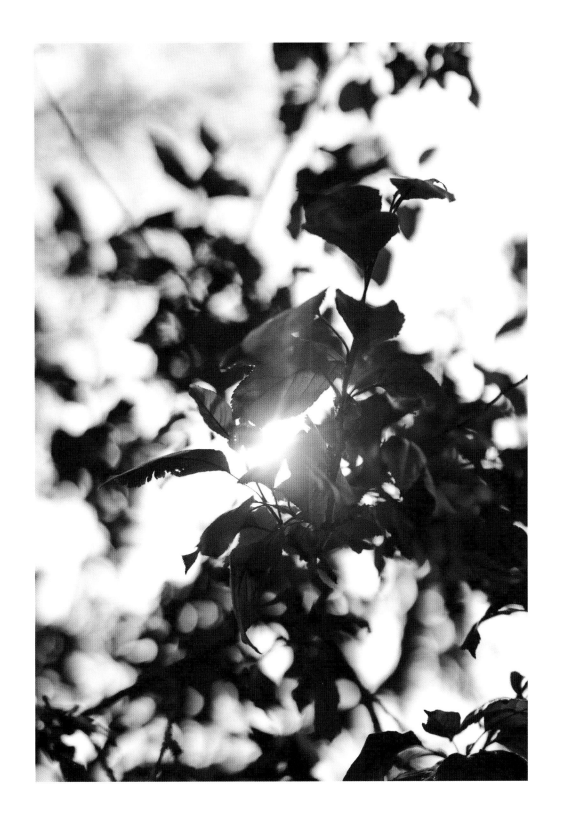

WAKING UP TO WHAT'S TYING YOU DOWN

When we're minimally reliant, we are maximally in control of our thoughts, feelings and behaviors. But before we can reduce our reliances, we first have to discover what they are. This means developing our powers of insight. Humans are complex creatures and the number of reliances we can have is effectively infinite. But I have identified eight major reliances, each of which seriously impacts a large number of people, and often remains invisible to them. Each chapter of *Make Change That Lasts* is a deep exploration of one of these major reliances. We're going to examine our need for other people to like us and validate our opinions. We'll break down our hidden attachment to myths we buy into about the heroes we look up to and measure ourselves against, and the false idea that our past controls our future. We're also going to analyze our reliance on comfort and success. We'll explore where these reliances – and a great many more – come from and learn to identify them in ourselves.

Once our hidden reliances have been identified, we will discover how to break free of them. Simply becoming aware of our reliances and understanding the power they exert over our lives will immediately change our relationship to them. And because

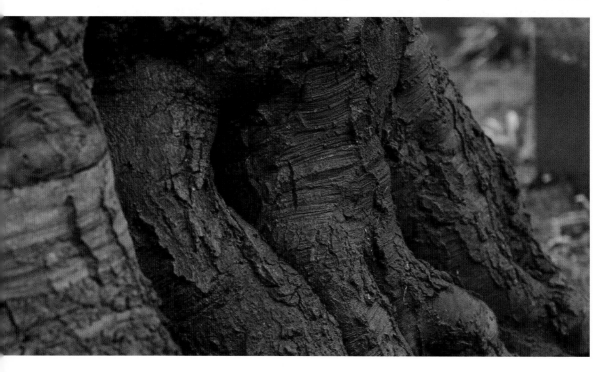

we are now conscious of the invisible forces that have been influencing the way we feel and act, we are better able to live more intentionally and make purposeful choices that are aligned with who we want to be.

THE THRIVE SIGNAL

Each chapter of this book contains small and easy practices that will help you become aware of your hidden reliances and reduce your dependency on them. The practices are so effective that you're likely to feel the benefits within a week. It's my experience that just moving the dial slightly will be enough for you to begin feeling like a different, more powerful version of yourself.

This is partly because of how your brain works. Your subconscious mind is continually looking for signals that tell it how your life is going. If it receives signals that indicate things are out of control and that you're struggling, the brain will alter its settings. Some of these settings are physical: it will move you into an unhealthy "stress state." Other settings are emotional: the brain will try to warn you that things aren't good by making you feel anxious, depressed or overly sensitive and reactive. All of these negative settings make it more likely that you will reach for the comfort of your unhealthy habits.

Just by starting the process of cutting your invisible needs and expectations, you will replace your stress signal with a thrive signal. Your brain will realize things are coming under control – and under control is exactly how you will begin to feel. There's a huge amount of scientific research that shows that people who have an increased sense of control are happier, have more money, better relationships and improved mental and physical health. The benefits are vast, and you will receive them on top of the benefits you'll get from eliminating those unhealthy habits that have previously always been so hard to quit. Minimal Reliance is the ultimate double win.

I don't think there's a single part of your life that won't improve for the better when you become minimally reliant. It will benefit you physically, making you stronger, healthier and extending your life. It will benefit you psychologically, making you calmer, less anxious and more confident, resilient and capable. It will give you new powers of control over your unhealthy behaviors. And the more you engage with the practices within the book, the more dramatic these changes will be. It won't just transform *your* life, it will even touch the lives of the people around you. Your family, friends and workmates will appreciate the new version of you that has more to give and is a positive force to be around.

MINIMAL NOT ZERO

Minimal Reliance isn't about never allowing ourselves to have a sugary treat, an alcoholic drink or a period of vulnerability. It's about growing ourselves physically and mentally so that we can *choose* when we do so. The state we're pursuing is not one of never being able to enjoy an indulgent dessert or the odd glass of wine; it's about building up our resilience so that we don't need to use these comforts as crutches but, instead, can engage with them intentionally.

It's also important to note that, like everything, the concept of Minimal Reliance can be taken too far. As we'll explore in the final chapter of this book, humans are highly social animals who have evolved to thrive in the context of a connected group. A certain amount of reliance is a basic fact of human life. The exercises I've designed and the philosophy I've described in these pages will ensure that you're the kind of person who gives to your groups – whether they be family, work or friendship circles – more than you expect in return. But healthy connection to a group is not only about us providing support for others. We also need others to provide support for us. Having people in our lives who we can rely on is a crucial ingredient for living a happy and healthy life. The goal we are aiming for is minimal reliance, not zero reliance.

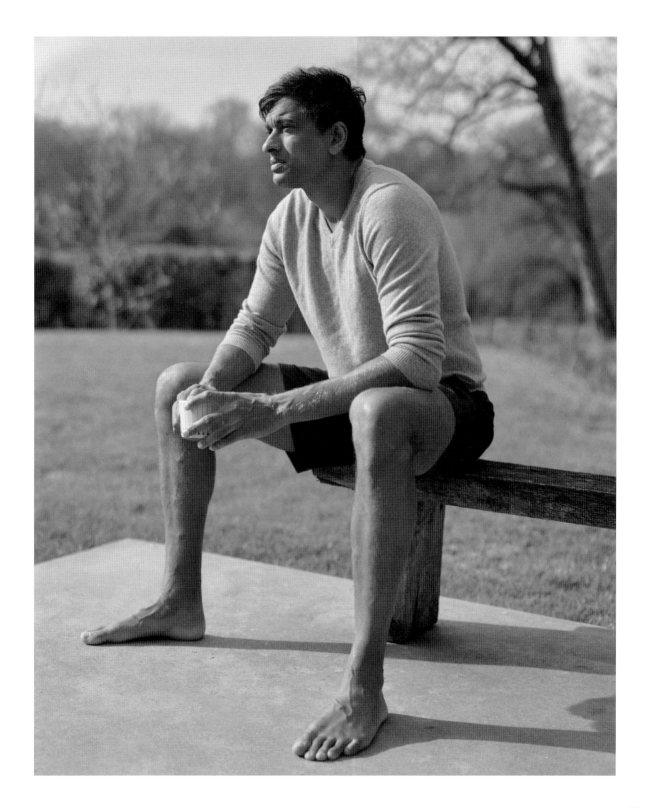

THE MAXIMAL POWER OF MINIMAL RELIANCE

I know how well this philosophy works because I have been following it myself for the past few years and have experienced its transformative effects. It has also helped numerous patients of mine. Perhaps best of all, it's helped the person who initially got me thinking about reliances. I spent many hours with Helen, trying to understand the stresses that were causing her to lose control of her eating behavior. It soon became apparent that one of the things people admired in her, and that she admired in herself, was, in fact, the hidden upstream cause of her sugar habit.

Helen hated complaining – especially to her colleagues at work. She loved serving people and being a doctor and believed that it was part of her duty to just suck up all the stresses and strains of the GP life, no matter what. Of course, this made her extremely popular, in particular with the person in charge of her practice, who would always turn to her to cover shifts when other GPs were out sick. The truth was, Helen was exhausted. And, privately, she resented always having to take up the slack for everyone else. She felt exploited and unappreciated; she'd come home and complain to her husband, but she'd never say a thing at work.

After spending a few weeks identifying exactly what triggered her to head to the newsagent's chocolate shelf, Helen realized it was when she felt tired or exploited or taken for granted. We also spent a lot of time discussing why she felt unable to speak up for herself and she soon realized she had an invisible reliance on being liked by everyone caused, in part, by a period of bullying she'd experienced at school. It was only when she let go of this reliance, and risked rejection by creating some boundaries with her boss, that she was able to finally take control of her snacking.

One of the most impactful things I advised Helen to do was to practice catching herself whenever she felt tempted to buy chocolate and take a moment to "look upstream." This became a kind of mantra for her. Every time she felt like she was going to crumble, she'd tell herself to "look upstream" at the cause of her discomfort. After a while, she didn't have to repeat these words. It happened automatically. She didn't have to try to control her behavior any more. It became effortless.

If you've bought this book because you're struggling with a stubborn habit, this is what you can achieve by developing your insight and reducing the number of reliances that you have. Effortless change is the best change of all. It's change that is automatic because it has become part of you.

Even if you're not struggling with a particular habit, this book truly has the power to transform your life. You can see Minimal Reliance as a philosophy for life. It will enable you to make sustainable changes in all aspects of your life and improve your mental health, physical health and your relationships. Many of my patients report it's even made them more successful: people they work with just want to be around them more. Those on the path of Minimal Reliance have this incredible magnetism. They look in control. They feel in control. They are in control. And who wouldn't want that?

"Effortless change is the best change of all. It's change that is automatic because it has become part of you."

1. TRUST YOURSELF

Reliance on experts

The day I said goodbye to my dad for the last time, I learned a powerful lesson. He'd been ill for fifteen years with an autoimmune condition called lupus and taking care of him had become a huge part of my life. There were many occasions during his illness when I would wake up at 5 a.m., drive around to his house, get him out of bed, help him dress, shave him and give him breakfast. I'd then dash back home briefly before shooting off to my GP practice. I'd use my lunch hour to go back and check in on him again. After four or five hours of seeing patients, I'd go to see him for a final time. And when he was at Manchester Royal Infirmary, I'd drive all the way into the city to visit him two or three times a day.

If Dad ever needed anything at all, giving it to him became the most important thing in my life. I put his care above everything else – my wife, my work, my health. I absolutely believed that the job of managing his needs was all on me. The crazy thing is that this was a purely self-generated idea. My mum and my brother didn't think that caring for Dad fell entirely on my shoulders. But, for some reason, looking after him became a massive part of my identity. When I failed, my failure became a reflection of who I was. One day his consultant surprised me by saying, "We've never seen anyone do so much for one person before." When he died in 2013, I was devastated. It was the first time I'd ever had to deal with the death of someone really close to me, and I honestly struggled to cope.

For a long time, including during Dad's illness, I'd been battling serious back pain. I'd spent thousands of pounds on various specialists, most of whom weren't able to help me all that much. I eventually found an expert in human movement and anatomy named Gary Ward, who helped me improve things significantly. But the discomfort

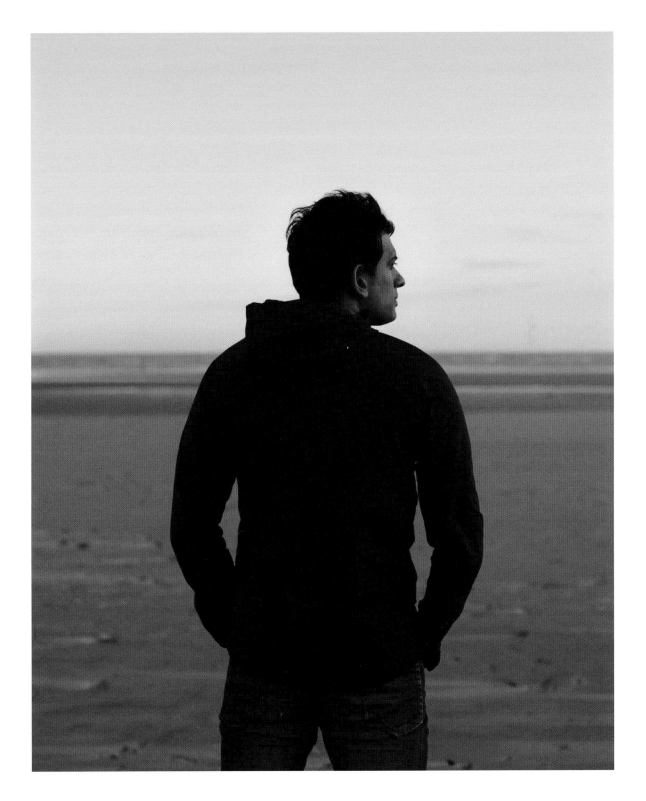

never completely lifted. Yes, I could get back to doing many of the things I'd previously had to give up, like playing squash, and I was able to sit pain-free for long car rides. But I was often aware of a lingering tightness in the right part of my lower back.

I had known for years that emotions could manifest as physical symptoms, but I never fully grasped the concept until the day of Dad's funeral. I dressed up in my best suit for the beautiful ceremony that was held at Manchester Crematorium, and played a song called "Tell Me Why" that I'd written for him a few years back, after he had dropped me off at university. Towards the end of the funeral, just before the actual cremation took place, I did everything I could to keep myself together. Then the black curtains opened and I glimpsed the furnace. As the coffin moved towards the fire, Dad's death suddenly became real. Up until that point I hadn't really absorbed the fact that I'd never have another conversation again with him again. This man that I loved, and who taught me how to play ping-pong and snooker; this person I used to follow around like a faithful dog while he was mowing the lawn on Saturday afternoons, was, right at that moment, being reduced to ashes.

Then something unexpected happened. When I saw the coffin start to go into the orange flames and heat, all the remaining pain in my back vanished. I realized that the discomfort was all the pressure I'd been holding in my body. It was literally the weight of expectation I'd been putting on myself. The simple knowledge that Dad was gone hadn't been enough to make the pain lift from my back – it took the sight of his body being burned into ashes for my subconscious to fully take in the message, you don't have to look after him any more.

That pain was a signal from my body that I wasn't thriving. My system had been telling me that it was struggling, but its message had been completely lost on me. I'd been unable to interpret the language of my own body. I've often explained to patients that the signals our bodies emit are a bit like birdsong. Most of the time, when we're walking down the street and the birds are singing, we block out their music. We're so busy getting on with our lives that we generally don't hear it. And even when we do notice the sound, we lack the ability to interpret what it means. If we're going to live a life of thriving, it's essential that we learn to hear and understand the music of our bodies.

When we're overly reliant on things outside of us, and being held down by wants, wishes and needs, the body will often let us know. When I look back now to the time

I used to care for Dad, I don't regret a thing. However, on reflection, my belief that his wellbeing was entirely my responsibility wasn't helpful. The truth was, he had a loving family and a brilliant team of medical professionals all available to him. But, for whatever reason, I generated a myth for myself to live by that said I could only be happy if I personally met his every need. That myth trapped me. It was the cause of a great deal of pain in my body and mind as well as to my wife, who had to deal with my regular absences and my significantly increased loads of stress. If I'd been able to hear my body's signals, I would have realized much earlier that something was wrong. If I knew then what I know now, I would have meditated on the issue, realized that this damaging myth was holding me down, and empowered myself to make changes.

THE EXPLOSION OF EXPERTS

One reason we can find it hard to listen to our own signals is that we're deafened by a bombardment of messages from the outside world. This is increasingly true in the age of the internet and social media. Don't get me wrong: I realize these technologies have been wonderful for people in many ways; I myself rely on them to reach a large number of people around the world, who listen to my podcasts and follow me on Instagram and other social platforms. But it's probably not going to be news to you that I also worry that online tech is also the cause of a lot of problems in peoples' wider lives.

One issue I've seen up close too many times to count is that social media encourages an unhealthy over-reliance on other peoples' opinions. Of course, it's human nature to seek out authority figures who can teach us useful lessons. We're subconsciously programmed to identify those people who seem to know what they're talking about and learn what we can from them. For the hundreds of thousands of years that we survived without the internet, these processes worked pretty well. The experts we gravitated towards might have been elder members of our hunter-gatherer tribes or professors in universities or talking heads on television or in newspapers – people that usually had some qualification that earned them their platform. But social media has led to an explosion of expertise. I'm not suggesting that people on the internet don't know what they're talking about – many are incredibly smart and well worth listening to. And there is no question that the internet has enabled more people to have a voice from a variety of different backgrounds – and that diversity is clearly a good thing. The problem I'm interested in here isn't their ability, it's that there are simply too many of them. We evolved to survive and thrive in mobile tribes in which there would be a small number of people we could learn from. Today there are thousands of voices we can tune into in an instant, each one confident, informed and apparently useful – and often insisting that the expert you've just been listening to, who seemed just as sure of themselves, is actually completely wrong.

The particular problem with being overly reliant on health and wellbeing experts is that what might be true for one person might not necessarily be true for the next. Every single one of us is completely unique, with different strengths and weaknesses. We vary in our genes, our microbiota, our physical and mental experience and our trauma. Just as no two minds are the same, no two digestive systems, muscular systems, immune systems, metabolic systems and neuroendocrine systems are the same. This means that the same piece of advice may not be suitable for everyone. For some of you, a plant-based diet may well be optimal and have the best health-enhancing effects, at the particular time in your life that you happen to be trying it. Others might thrive on the paleo diet or one containing large amounts of meat and fish. For others, intermittent fasting is a game changer for their weight, energy and digestion. Others still might find this makes them moody and sluggish. Some people think that their yoga practice is the best thing that ever happened to them, and become evangelical about it, insisting that everyone on the planet would be better off if they just started doing it themselves. But guess what? You don't have to do yoga – or anything else any expert insists you have to do.

In fact, continuing to follow a plan that is not suiting you or your lifestyle in the hope that you'll be healthy and happy when you've lost a certain amount of weight or run a 10K or whatever else you might be hoping for, is actually incredibly harmful and creates a huge amount of stress inside your body. In addition, when you have outsourced your own expertise about your own body to someone else and when their expertise is not yielding results, it can often lead to disappointment. More often than not, we feel worse than if we had never taken that expert's advice in the first place, because we feel that there is something wrong with us. The expert had the "perfect" advice, but we were the ones unable to act on it and realize the benefits.

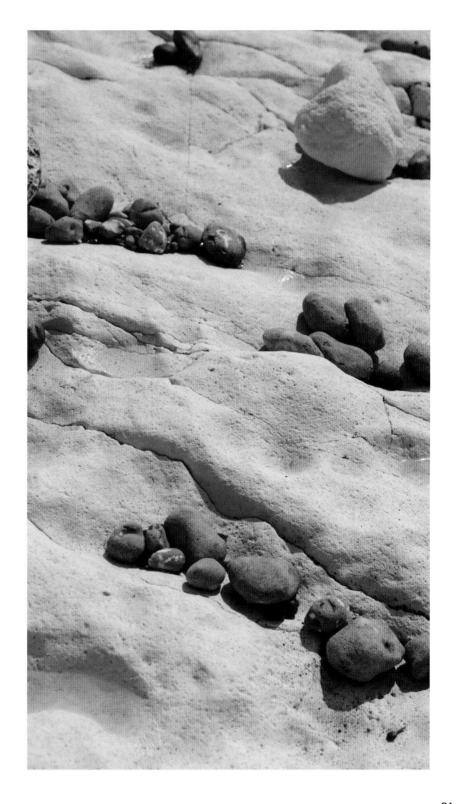

"You don't have to do yoga – or anything else any expert insists you have to do."

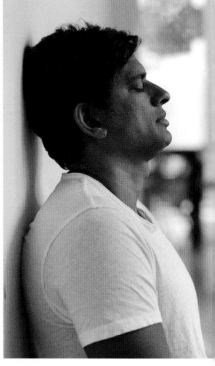

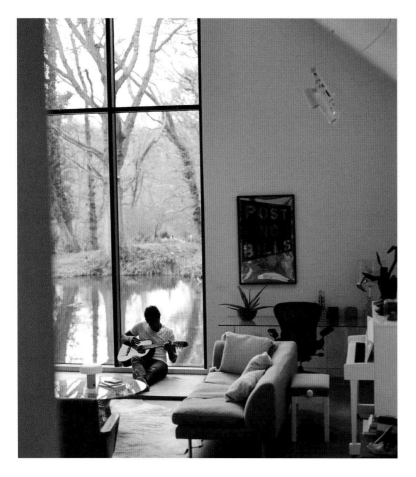

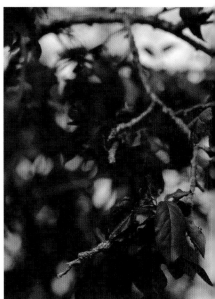

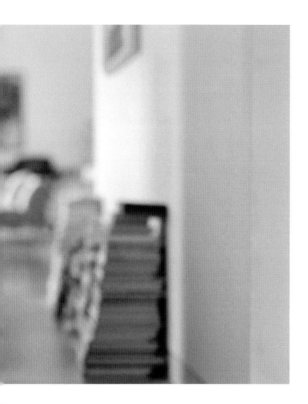

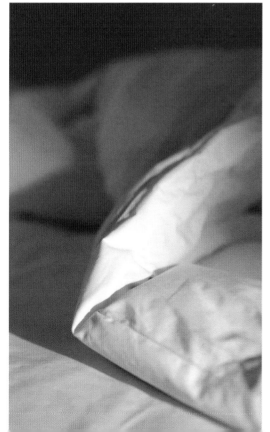

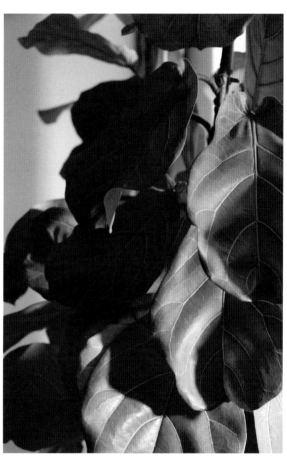

Sometimes, simply reading the advice of experts can have negative consequences if we are not secure enough in who we are and the life choices that we are making. I once saw a middle-aged mother of four in my practice who was devastated after reading in a popular British newspaper that spouses that had sex less than ten times a year were officially in a "sexless marriage." She told me that she and her husband were happy and just didn't feel a particular need, in their late forties, to have sex all that often. But that newspaper story had led to her feeling as if she was failing. She and her husband had begun doubting their relationship. They had begun comparing themselves to a fantasy ideal marriage that wasn't actually relevant to them. Reading the advice from that "sex expert" had done real harm to her marriage and her self-image.

While it can be helpful to look to experts for answers and to discuss the problems in our lives with other people, this should ultimately help us become *less* reliant on others as we build up our own inner awareness. When we outsource our wellbeing to other people, we forget that not only are we different from the next person, but also that we carry within us a lifetime's worth of learning and experience that's highly specialized to our own unique minds and bodies.

CASE STUDY

I once saw a 54-year-old lady who came in to see me as she was struggling with her digestion. She was an avid consumer of health information online and had developed a real interest in gut health. She had read that eating thirty different plants each week would help her and she'd been trying to introduce this into her life for months. Every time she increased the amount of plant foods in her diet – whether gradually or not – she would experience unpleasant symptoms such as bloating, abdominal discomfort and constipation. She beat herself up for months thinking that she was "doing it wrong" and couldn't figure out why it was not working. At the same time, she was reading about other people who managed to do it just fine and were feeling better. She felt frustrated and created a lot of internal stress for herself by believing that she was failing. When she came in to see me, I explained that not every bit of advice – no matter how good – works for every single individual and that the most important thing for us all is to figure out what works for us. Over time, she decided to follow a more "low-carb" style of eating with, perhaps, only five to ten different plant foods each week. When she ate in this fashion, she thrived. Her digestion improved, her sleep was much better and she experienced more energy and vitality than she had in years. Her blood tests looked great as well. She had discovered what worked for her.

WHY I'VE NEVER TOLD A PATIENT THEY MUST QUIT SMOKING

I've always managed to cultivate good relationships with the vast majority of my patients and, more often than not, helped them make sustainable changes to their lives. I think one of the main reasons for that is that I've always treated them as equals. If a smoker came in asking for help, I would explain the impact their habit is having on them and recommend that they think about giving up cigarettes. But if, after our chat, I was happy that they had clearly understood me and they said, "Doc, I understand. But, for me, I get so much enjoyment out of smoking, I am happy to put up with the consequences," then I would respect their decision. They are adults. They are free to make their own choices, as we all are.

I'd even extend this argument to the book that's in your hands right now. If you disagree with something in it, I say "good." I don't want you to be overly reliant on me and my opinion, and to follow it without question. But, equally, I'm not suggesting that you completely ignore me or any other expert when it comes to good advice that might help you. I've spent my adult life learning from brilliant people, and I don't intend to stop anytime soon.

So how do you strike the right balance? The best way of navigating this galaxy of experts is to hear them out, absorb their messaging and then ask yourself which message feels right to you. Which one resonates? Which gives you a feeling of excitement and possibility? Which "rings true?" This is the expert I'd recommend you prioritize, as these feelings are from your subconscious: something deep inside you is communicating with you, trying to get you to pay attention to them. Then, experiment. Use yourself as data. Try out their recommendations. Journal how you feel each day. In this way you will become a world expert in you.

OVER-RELIANCE ON THE HEAD

Another way of putting it is like this: learn to listen to your gut and start trusting it a bit more. In the West, we have a head-driven culture, where we think we can explain and rationalize everything with our minds. We ignore the fact that some of the deepest intelligence we have, as humans, is located deep within our bodies.

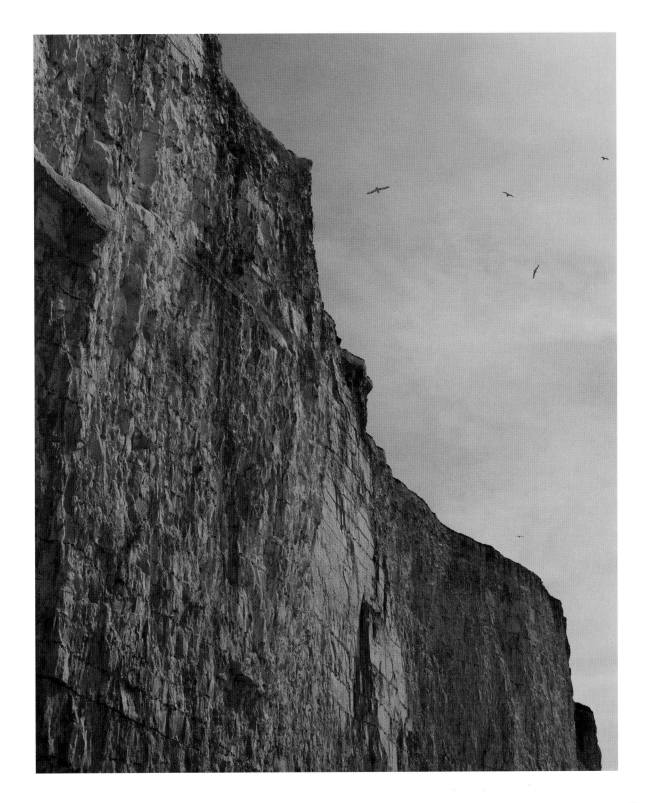

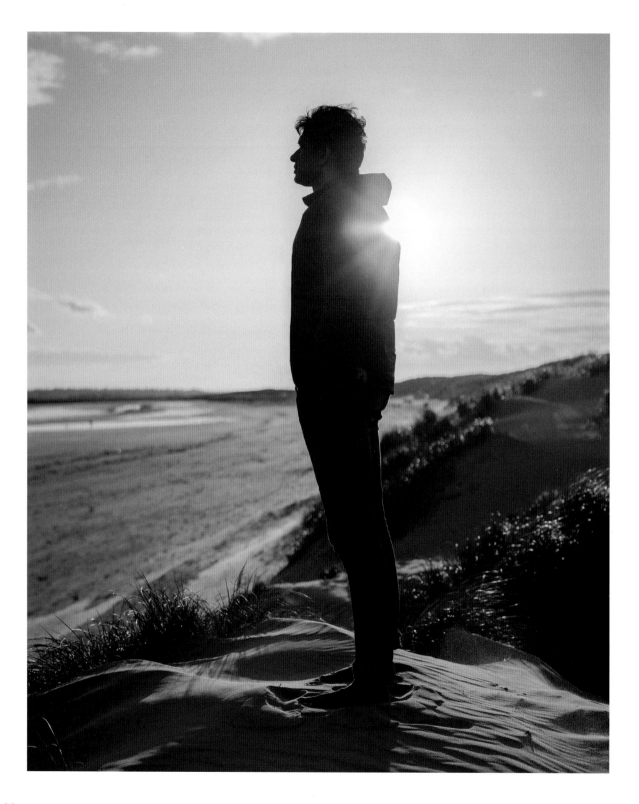

I'll never forget reading an account of the Zen master D. T. Suzuki describing the visit of an American scientist to an aboriginal tribe. When the scientist explained that his fellow countrymen thought with their heads, the people in the tribe were confused. They thought the Americans must be crazy. They explained, "We think with our abdomens." I felt this was such a telling comment. I truly believe that there is an innate wisdom in our bodies, one that many of us have lost touch with. Learning to tap into it is a key skill in the journey to becoming more aware of our reliances in the outside world and making intentional decisions based on an enhanced understanding of ourselves.

The latest research certainly backs up what these Aboriginal people were saying. Scientists are indeed learning that our bodies are astonishingly deep sources of information, if only we can learn to listen to them properly. One of the most exciting and rapidly growing new fields is the study of what's known as "interoception." Interoception is literally a sixth sense – like sight, touch, taste, sound and smell, it's a basic power of detection that we're born with. But interoception doesn't interpret signals from the outside world. Instead, it's directed inward at the signals that are transmitted from our internal organs to our brains. Probably the most well-known interoceptive signal is our heartbeat; we've all read those thrillers that use a character's rapid heart rate as a shorthand for showing they are under pressure and feeling scared or stressed. But it turns out it's not just the heart that gives out information as to what's going on with us, but the entire functioning body. Everything from our gut to our bladder to our lungs, muscles, kidneys and cardiovascular system is continually talking to our brains. And the better we get at listening to its messages, the better able we are to thrive.

A large number of recent scientific studies suggest that an improved sense of interoception can transform our wellbeing. For example, a study published in *The Lancet* reported on research done by Professor Hugo Critchley at the Brighton and Sussex Medical School with autistic individuals who had symptoms of anxiety. Professor Critchley was able to significantly reduce their stress levels by training them to be more aware of signals from their heartbeats. After just six sessions, 31 percent of them recovered completely from their anxiety compared to only 16 percent in the control group. Professor Cynthia Price at the University of Washington in Seattle has carried out equally impressive work with people who have substance abuse problems. Drug and alcohol addicts who relapse often struggle to regulate their emotions; Price found that training patients to be more acutely aware of their internal sensations, with sessions of mindfulness that were focused inward, lessened their cravings, reduced depression and helped them remain abstinent over the course of a year.

Given that improved interoception does so much good for people battling anxiety and dependency, you'd rightly assume that it can work wonders for everyone else. In fact, some researchers believe that one of the reasons physical exercise can reduce symptoms of anxiety and depression is because of increased interoceptive awareness. By regularly increasing our heart rate and working out our muscles, we become more attuned to the signals our bodies are emitting, which in turn helps us feel more capable and in control.

THE TROUBLE WITH TRACKERS

Given how much I'm emphasizing the importance of self-knowledge to thriving, you might assume that I'd be a huge fan of health trackers that give us a wealth of individualized personalized data, from how many steps we're taking each day to how well we're sleeping. But the current trend for tracking every aspect of our lives, without the necessary knowledge to interpret what we find, is fraught with potential problems. Take sleep trackers. I used to use one of these to monitor my sleep each night. One morning I woke up feeling great and assumed that I'd slept pretty well. But when I checked my tracker sleep score on the device, it was low. This immediately began to play on my mind. One hour later, I began to feel sluggish and irritable. I couldn't help but wonder: was I actually tired? Or was the device on my wrist somehow changing my perception? Perhaps seeing the score on my tracker had sent a negative signal to my brain, and it was that that was dragging down my wellbeing?

A couple of scientific studies that have taken place more recently have supported my suspicions. In the first study, two groups of subjects slept in a lab for either five hours or eight hours. When they woke up, the group who had slept five hours were told they had actually slept eight hours and vice versa. The researchers found that those who'd slept five hours, but believed they'd had a full night's rest, did not feel bad. But the other group, who'd slept well but were told they hadn't, had worse cognitive performance. A second study, carried out by researchers at Stanford University, found that when people were told (untruthfully) that their daily step counts were low, they consequently ate less healthily, experienced more negative emotions, had reduced self-esteem and increased blood pressure and heart rate.

These studies tell me that trackers have the potential to create a powerful reliance in many people that negatively affects their ability to thrive. Some people who use them find that they can only feel good about themselves when the number on their screen has good news to report back to us. Many of them are also, by their very nature, extremely reductionist, reducing our complex and multifaceted lives down into a stark and simple number. If the number is good, we are good. If the number is bad, we are bad. In addition, many of them do not help us make the crucial connection between the numbers that are being measured and the emotions that we are feeling. We will never thrive if we make our tracker scores a reliance. As the legendary physicist Albert Einstein said, "Not everything we measure matters. And not everything that matters can be measured."

But, as with all things, the truth about trackers doesn't lie at the extremes. For some people, they can be incredibly helpful if used mindfully and intentionally. Take continuous glucose monitors, for example. These CGMs can provide information that's almost impossible to get from any other source, helping us to understand how our bodies react to certain foods. Rather than being a constant guide to how we're doing in the game of life, they teach us information about ourselves that we can use when the tracker itself has been put back in the drawer. We all respond differently to different foods and knowing which kinds of foods give us significant blood glucose spikes can be very useful. If we learn that when we eat pizza our blood glucose goes into the diabetic range, that is powerful information to have, information that – perhaps – will help us reduce our intake. If we learn that the sweet potato wedges we are eating five times a week because we think they are "healthy" are causing us to have a huge glucose crash two to three hours later, which is also the exact time when we feel moody, tired and hungry, then we'll be able to make more empowered choices going forward. At this point in my life, I personally use a CGM for two weeks, maybe two or three times a year, simply as a way to check up and keep me on track with my food choices. Doing it this way means that the information it gives me empowers me, rather than tying me down.

Your job is to find out what works for you. Health trackers are simply a tool and, like all tools, they can be helpful or harmful depending on how they are used. If you use them for a specific purpose, for discrete periods of time, in order to help you

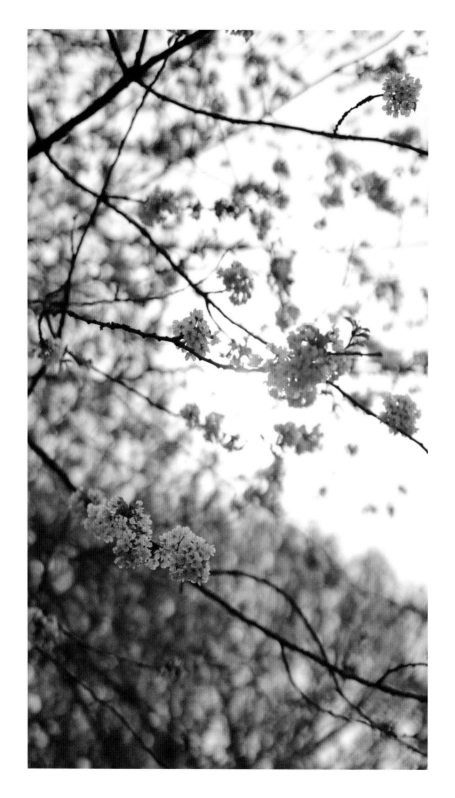

understand yourself better, they can absolutely be powerful tools for change. But if you are becoming overly obsessed with the data, are unable to function without them and they're negatively affecting the way you view yourself and your experience of everyday life, they're likely to be harming you instead of empowering you.

YOUR INNER BAROMETER

Rather than relying on technology or experts to tell us how to feel, we should learn to rely mostly on ourselves. This means approaching both our health and our wider life with a spirit of playful curiosity. We should start to see our lives as an adventure of constant exploration. We are all on a journey of learning about ourselves that won't end until the day we die. And each of our journeys are different. As we continue this journey of discovery, we should remember that even the world's most reputable experts will inevitably be wrong about some things. When I arrived at medical school, I was told that 50 percent of what we would be taught would end up being wrong, we just didn't know which 50 percent. There is so much that we don't know. All we can ever do is make the best decisions we can, based on our practiced expertise in ourselves.

That expertise will come when we learn to truly listen to our brains and bodies. I have a close friend who's a keen practitioner of yoga. When he's going through his morning routine, he knows if his stress load is rising and starting to negatively affect him because, rather than being fluid and easy, his Sun Salutation sequence feels rigid and uncomfortable. He sees this as his inner barometer. It's the tell – from his body – that he needs to take extra care of himself that day. My inner barometer is my daily breathing exercise. Sometimes I can hold my breath for a minute less than other times. When this happens, I take it as a signal that something in my life needs addressing and then meditate on it, using one of the exercises below. I try to understand – what is going wrong for me? What is it in my life that's holding me back? What is keeping me from being free?

A common barometer for many people is irritation and impatience. We often assume that our bad moods cause bodily sensations such as high blood pressure and elevated heart rate. But, sometimes, it might be the case that the signals from our bodies are causing these moods, not the other way around. If, for example, we find ourselves getting irritated or lashing out at other people, it might be that we are responding not to the person in front of us, but to the signals our body is emitting.

CREATING TIME FOR SOLITUDE

Regular time spent intentionally alone is of critical importance to thriving. Like a piano that has been left to go out of tune, our brains and bodies will become discordant if we don't take a quiet moment to listen to them with focused concentration, and then make the necessary adjustments. I would really encourage you to block off some time each day with the specific intention of connecting with yourself. In my experience, first thing in the morning works best for most people, as a practice at this time can set the tone for the rest of your day. However, I appreciate that we all lead unique lives with different pressures and so, consistent with the theme of this chapter, you will have to experiment and discover what works best for you. However, please don't fall into the common trap of thinking you don't have time for this crucially important practice – even 5 or 10 minutes will make a huge difference.

There are a variety of practices that you could consider introducing into your life, to help you get to know yourself better. Here are some examples to get you thinking but feel free to come up with your own:

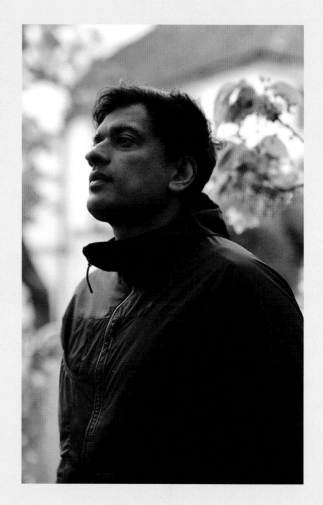

MEDITATION

One of my favorite solitude practices is meditation. There are many ways to meditate but one technique that helps us develop better self-awareness is doing a type of body scan. At the same time every day, sit in silence while placing your focus on the inner body, starting at the toes and working your way upward, slowly and carefully, to the top of the head. Some days, the practice will feel free and fluid. Other days, you may feel tension in certain parts of

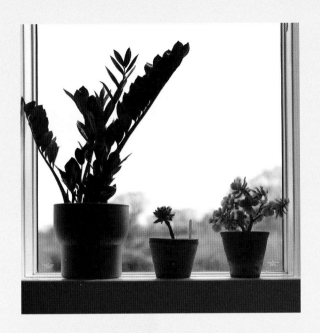

your body as well as a barrage of internal chaos. When you feel chaotic and stressed, it is critically important that you remember not to judge yourself: you are simply observing what is going on with you on that particular day. That is how you cultivate the skill. You are not actually looking for calm every single day because that is not realistic. What you feel will change from day to day because life is constantly changing. The goal is to get to know yourself and observe what is happening. This allows you to make better decisions in every aspect of your life. The more you practice, the better you will get at noticing subtle differences in the body each day.

BREATHWORK

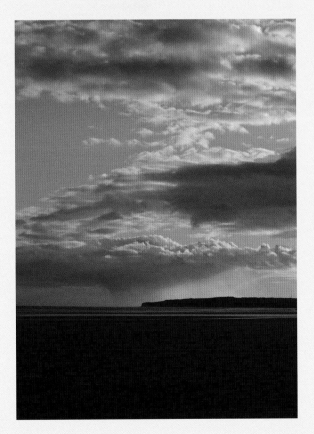

You could also do a similar practice with the focus being solely on your breath. Sit in silence and for 5 minutes or so, just pay attention to your breath. How does it feel? Are there any restrictions as you breathe in or out? Where does it feel free and fluid and where does it feel tight? Can you breathe into the tight areas and watch them loosen up? Does this change from day to day? There are many other breathwork practices that you could consider, such as my 3-4-5 breath, that I first wrote about in *The 4 Pillar Plan*. You simply breathe in for 3 seconds, hold your breath for 4 seconds and breathe out for 5 seconds, and repeat over and over again. Please don't fall into the trap of overcomplicating this. All you are looking for is a simple breathwork practice that helps you pay attention to what is going on inside your body.

YOGA

Yoga is another fantastic practice that you could consider that really helps develop awareness between body and mind. The word "yoga" literally means "union:" union of your mind, body and spirit. It has been practiced regularly for over five thousand years and, when done regularly, can help us pay attention to what is going on inside our bodies and develop our own internal self-awareness. It can also lower stress, improve sleep and reduce pain. A simple 5- or 10-minute practice each morning can work wonders.

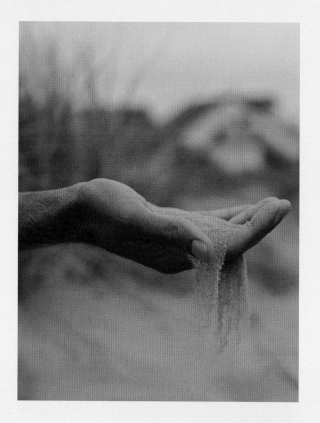

JOURNALING

Unlike daily solitude practices like body scanning, yoga and breathwork that help you build up your own awareness through your body, practices like journaling can help you develop self-awareness by using your brain. Both methods can be powerful depending on your preferences and, of course, it is possible to do both. I personally love to journal each morning for a few minutes after I complete my meditation. I find that meditation opens a door in my mind to enable me to discover fresh insights about myself. I then crystallize those insights by journaling immediately afterward. There are many different methods of journaling out there for you to experiment with and it's important to experiment and find out what works best for you. My own favorite is to ask myself a few powerful questions each morning, which help me learn, reflect and grow. You can read more about my own favorite questions in my book *The Three Question Journal* or by listening to my podcast episode at drchatterjee.com/413.

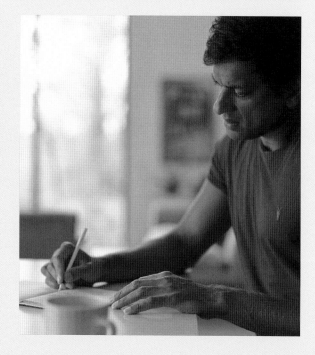

There is no one "right way" to develop the skill of listening to your body. All you are looking for is a daily practice that you can commit to. And it's important to remember that *doing* a solitude practice regularly is much more important than trying to figure out the "perfect" practice that you only manage to engage with from time to time!

Whichever practice you choose, it is a good idea to do the same one, every day, ideally at the same time. The magic lies in the repetition. When we repeat a practice over and over again, we quickly build up our innate intelligence and intuition.

We quickly learn to realize what is normal for us and recognize when things feel different. With consistent practice, we become our own expert, and reduce our reliance on the barrage of contradictory and confusing voices that surround us every day.

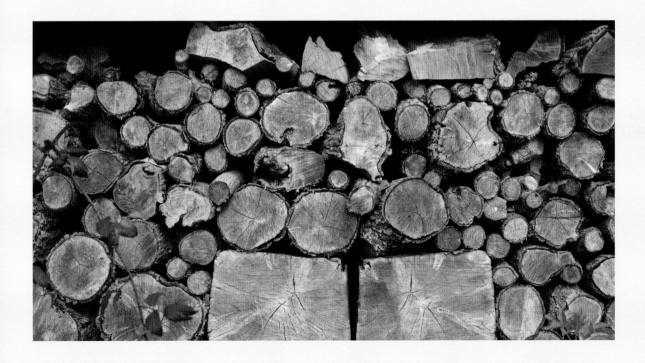

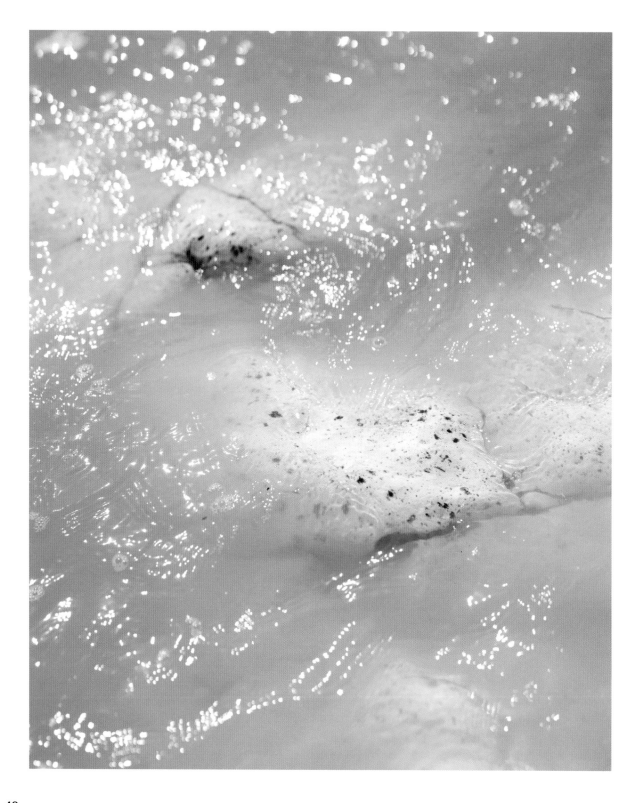

CONCLUSION

▶ Don't outsource your life to others. We are living through an explosion of expertise. Not all of these experts will have the right advice for everyone. We are all unique and the same piece of advice may not be suitable for everyone.

▶ Choose your experts by assessing how they make you feel. Listen to and think with your gut. Go with the advice that rings true. Use yourself as data: if something works, go with it; if not, empower yourself to try someone and something else.

▶ Develop your powers of insight by using solitude practices. Use them to learn the skill of listening to the messages your body is sending you. Over time, you will become much more aware of when your body is letting you know that something in your life needs addressing; for example, your work-load may be escalating beyond your capacity to cope or a close relationship in your life may be in need of some attention.

▶ Embrace the journey of becoming a world expert in you. As you get to know yourself better, you will become less susceptible to outside voices and more trusting of your own inner wisdom. This will have incredible downstream effects on your behaviors; you will feel more in control of yourself, less susceptible to unhealthy habits and better able to make positive changes that last.

2. GIVE UP YOUR HEROES

Reliance on perfection

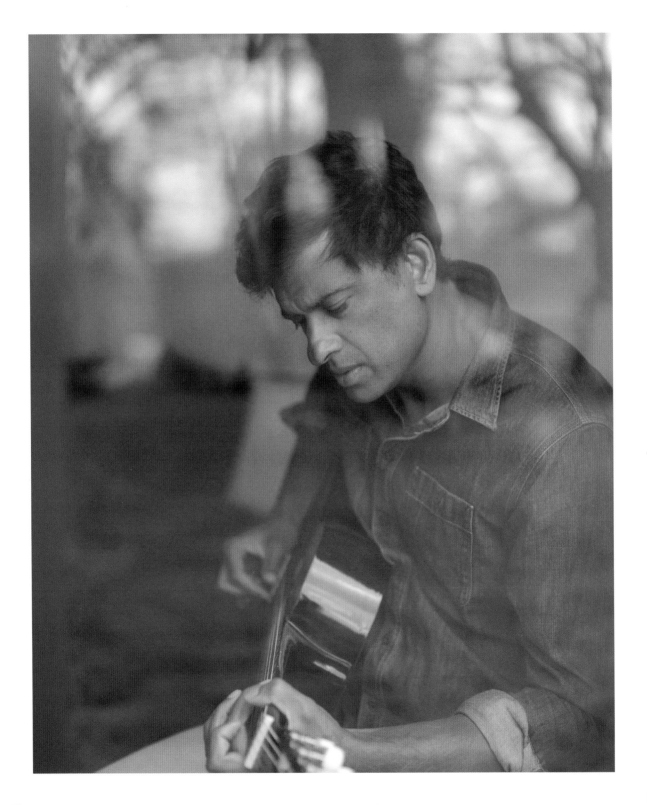

When I was a teenager, I wanted to be Jon Bon Jovi. My bedroom walls were covered in posters of the singer and his band, and one of my prized possessions was a huge silk Bon Jovi flag that I had pinned up next to my desk. I honestly thought that if I could be Jon Bon Jovi, my life would be perfect. I mean, what wasn't to like? He was successful, handsome, talented and wealthy. He had cool tattoos and hordes of screaming fans. He appeared to be constantly performing in stadiums all over the globe and he was the center of attention, wherever he went. To me, a typical teenage boy, the everyday life of Jon Bon Jovi sounded like heaven on earth.

The human ideal that my music idol stood for never left my imagination. In my subconscious mind, Jon Bon Jovi became the perfect person, a model to look up to and emulate. I taught myself to write songs. At the age of eighteen, as soon as I got to university, I started a band in which I wrote songs, sang lead vocals and played guitar. Then, at the age of twenty-six, I arranged time off from my job as a doctor to play with my band in the iconic ski town of Chamonix-Mont-Blanc, France. We stayed for the entire three-month winter ski season, playing five nights a week to packed venues filled with people, who'd scream and dance to our music. We'd even end our sets with the classic Bon Jovi hit, "Livin' on a Prayer." It was incredible. Everything I'd imagined for Jon Bon Jovi I began living, in real life, for myself. I even met a bona fide pop star who told me, "Wow, everyone seems to love you here. You're more famous in Chamonix than I am."

Needless to say, this didn't end up being a recipe for a perfect life. Although on the outside it looked as if I was having an amazing time, on the inside I was struggling.

The fact is, I was running away from my life. I was so insecure in who I was that I was literally trying to become someone else. I made a mistake that is all too human – a mistake that, if we're not conscious of it, we risk making throughout our lives. I fell for the myth of the hero.

THE MYTH OF THE HERO

It's human nature to put people on a pedestal. It's no exaggeration to say that we're born with an instinct to make heroes of others. The first idealized people we come into contact with are our parents. We are programmed to look up to them because, without their care and support, we simply cannot survive. As babies, toddlers and then children we're hardwired to mimic their behavior. We learn how to act, what to believe and how the world works by watching them closely, listening to what they have to say, and partly absorbing who they are. If we have siblings, we learn from them too. But then we hit adolescence, and our pool of model humans suddenly expands. We become less interested, and often outright contemptuous, of what our mums and dads believe, and instead look to sources outside of the family unit. We join a peer group, and teenage peer groups pretty much always have humans that they model – heroes that their members are desperate to emulate in every tiny detail, like I did with Jon Bon Jovi.

This process of looking up to our heroes in order to mold and perfect ourselves can be healthily formative. But it can also have serious dangers. What I didn't understand as a young man was that I was falling for a myth that had been created, in part, by a hugely powerful marketing machine. I'd seen my idol in music videos and TV interviews and taken what had been presented to me as the truth. What I couldn't see, and had never even considered, were what I now imagine to be all the negative aspects of his life: the often dull and repetitive touring life, the realities of sleeping on a bus every night with a bunch of noisy, smelly band and crew, the months away from the family, the enormous pressure of having to perform for thousands of fans night after night, and to keep writing and recording brilliant album after brilliant album, so that the hundreds of people whose livelihoods came to depend on my band succeeding could keep their jobs and pay their rent. I also couldn't see the parts of his life that perhaps weren't so impressive. I've got no clue what Jon Bon Jovi is like in real life, but we all have sides to our personalities that can be rough around the edges. All I ever saw was the handsome, happy, romantic, macho, carefree god of rock. In my head, he was perfect. It never occurred to me that "perfect" could be a myth.

YOUR HEROES ARE NOT WHO YOU THINK THEY ARE

What's true of Jon Bon Jovi is even more true of some of the other people I've looked up to as heroes in my life. Michael Phelps, the swimmer who won an astonishing twenty-eight Olympic Medals, also suffered from severe depression and has admitted he feels lucky to not have taken his own life. Golfer Tiger Woods, the winner of an astonishing fifteen majors, suffered from public humiliation, an addiction to painkillers, and the widely reported failure of his marriage. Jonny Wilkinson, the rugby union player whose drop goal famously won the match during the last minute of the Rugby World Cup Final, found himself crippled with mental health problems. The list goes on. People like these are worshipped by millions all over the world. But is their life what we want? Do we really want to be just like them?

The truth is, your heroes are probably not who you think they are – they're probably not even who you want to be. When we idolize people, we only see a partial glimpse of them. You'll have heard the phrase "never meet your heroes." Why do we say that? Because we know deep down there's a high chance we'll be disappointed by them. How many musicians, writers, football idols and movie stars find themselves accused of behavior that's considered unhealthy or immoral? We shouldn't be surprised when our favorite singers end up being broken people and having flaws: they wrote those heart-wrenching songs in the first place because of their internal struggle and pain. As they say, sorrow breeds the sweetest tunes.

The way these people have been presented to us is not real. Corporate interests understandably want to hide all the difficult edges of their personalities from us, and ensure we only ever see their highlights reel. But like everyone else, our heroes also have a failures reel they'd rather not think about. Tim Ferris's book *The 4-Hour Work Week* was a global smash hit, selling over 2 million copies, but not before it was rejected by publishers twenty-six times. Almost everyone who's succeeded on a high level has also failed on a high level. The problem is, we're rarely shown these failures.

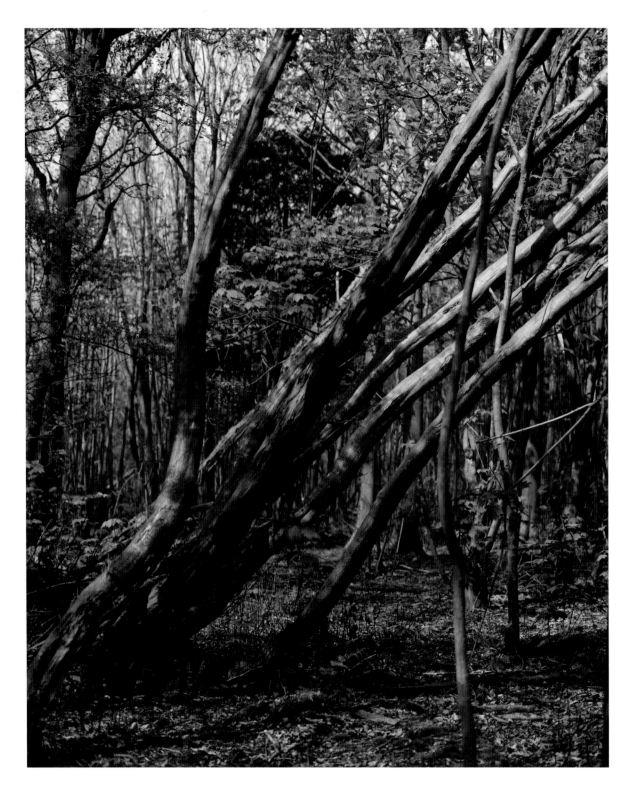

"It never occurred to me that 'perfect' could be a myth."

When we only look at the highlights reel, we can't help but feel inferior. In our low moments, we compare the worst version of ourselves to the best version of them. This is important because, when we feel "less than," we start to compensate. We might drink alcohol, binge on sugary snacks, stay up too late or experience chronic stress. We make ourselves sick by overworking and pushing ourselves beyond what we can cope with, in a futile attempt to live up to a fictional idea of "success" we've created inside our own heads. It's lifestyle factors like these that underpin 80–90 percent of all health complaints that are seen by doctors. What lies upstream from them are our thoughts about ourselves and the world. If these thoughts are toxic, our behaviors will be toxic as well.

"If our thoughts are toxic, our behaviors will be toxic as well."

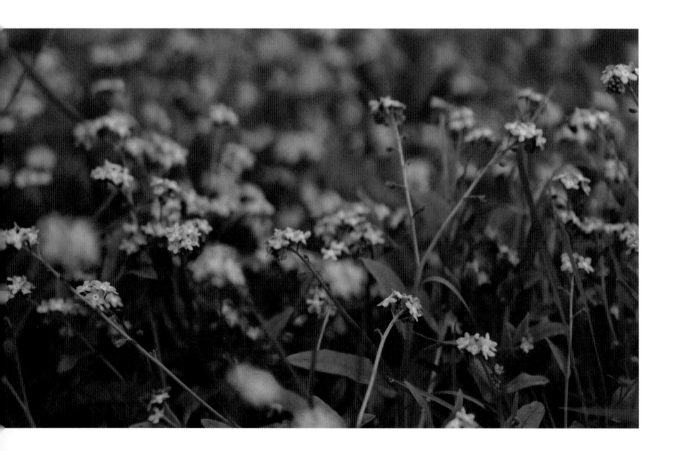

A PLAGUE OF PERFECTIONISM: WHEN HEROES HOLD US BACK

Some of the most toxic thoughts of all are perfectionistic, and perfectionism can be made much worse by hero-worship. In the modern world, we're utterly surrounded by heroes on television, film, the internet and billboards as we drive to work or wait on the platform for our train. Our attention is constantly being drawn towards spaces where there will be some picture of a person more beautiful and successful than we are. It didn't used to be like this; in the hunter-gatherer tribes we evolved from, there would probably have been only a handful of elders that we would have used as models to live by, and we would have been up close and personal to them, allowing us to become aware of their faults as well as their gifts. Today's endless river of polished and perfected singers, actors, models, writers and influencers make vast amounts of money and have huge machines around them, dedicated to making them seem as perfect as possible. But, in a very real sense, Jon Bon Jovi doesn't actually exist. Neither do any of today's heroes, be they Taylor Swift or Lionel Messi or Tiger Woods.

The "hero" figures presented to us are more like avatars, no more based in reality than cartoon characters. They're designed to trigger deep mechanisms that have evolved within us that make us want to look up to and mimic them, just as we did our parents when we were three years old. That's how the corporate machines around these figures make millions in profit. This has had a terrible effect on our mental health. Our subconscious models for what makes a good human have become impossible to achieve.

This is partly why psychologists have been raising the alarm about an increasing problem with perfectionism in many parts of the world – especially the West. A 2018 study of over 40,000 people in the US, UK and Canada found that levels of perfectionism had risen substantially. Between 1989 and 2016, the extent to which people felt they had to "display perfection to secure approval" had soared by an astonishing 33 percent. From an early age, we're surrounded by cultural heroes whose behavior and appearance literally changes the wiring of our brains, raising the bar as to what we consider to be acceptable for ourselves. We then stress ourselves out trying to reach this impossible bar.

Because many of these processes are subconscious, they can be hard to spot in our own behavior. But if you repeatedly feel like a failure – like you're "not good enough" in the eyes of others, or in your own judgement – then it's likely you're suffering from perfectionistic thinking. And, contrary to popular belief, being a perfectionist is not something to show off about in job interviews. It can be highly damaging to our mental and physical health, and plays a role in a host of disorders, including depression, self-harm, anorexia, bulimia and even suicidal thinking.

We can never thrive if our wellbeing has come to rely on us feeling like we're the same as the imaginary people we've put on a pedestal. We tend to think of "judging" other people as a matter of looking down our noses at them. But looking upward is judgement too, just in the other direction. No matter which direction we're looking in, judging others always comes from a fear of inadequacy inside ourselves. It's always based on simplifying and distorting the reality of other people and their lives in a way that's unhelpful. A huge part of achieving Minimal Reliance involves understanding the world as it actually is, not as how we imagine it to be. We'll never thrive if we make a habit of measuring our worth against our distorted fantasies of reality.

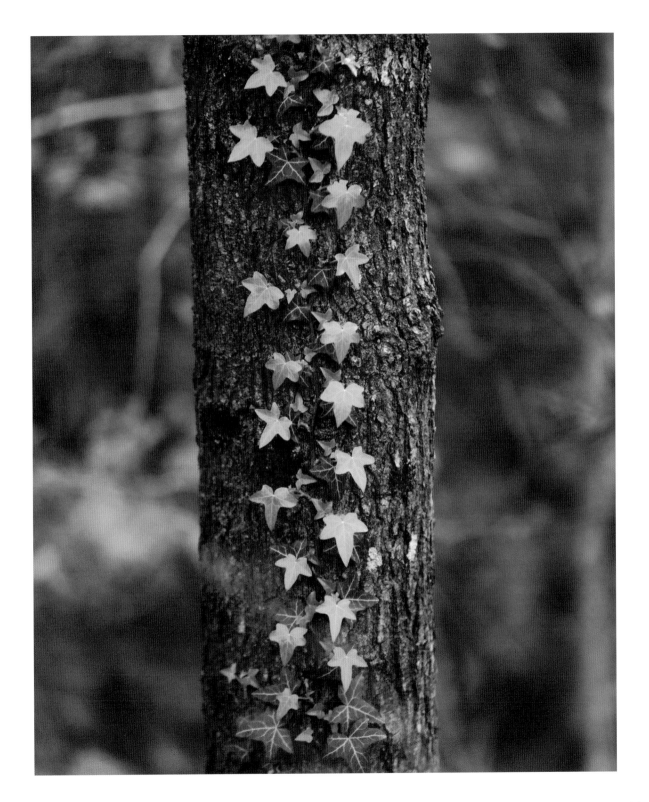

HAVING A HEALTHY RELATIONSHIP WITH HEROES

As ever, it's critical to remember that we always want to avoid the extremes. We're aiming for minimal – not zero – reliance. I would never advise anyone to shut out influence from other people completely. There is no question that many of our heroes can teach us valuable things and, of course, we should always be open to learning from them. The problem is that this often goes too far, and rather than just taking what's useful, we try to mimic the whole person – or rather our perception of the whole person – which is futile because we don't actually know them. When we do this, we sacrifice something sacred: our authenticity. It goes without saying that we'll never be the best version of ourselves if we're trying to be someone different. It's also worth remembering that many of your heroes didn't become your heroes by replicating their idols, but by pioneering their own path, and becoming well known and respected in their own right.

It's useful to meditate on why exactly you admire the people you do. There will be something in them that resonates powerfully with you, some quality or talent that you hope to develop yourself. I believe that when we recognize that thing in others, we're actually recognizing it in ourselves. Those people we look up to are chosen, by our subconscious

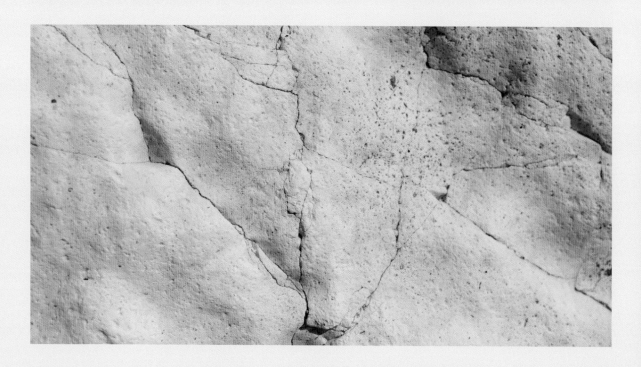

minds, for a reason. When we lock on to them, it's because our brain has detected in them a quality that we possess but needs to be developed. So make a practice of thinking about your heroes, and rather than worshipping everything about them, isolate exactly what quality they embody that you also have in a smaller quantity. Is it their courage? Their grit? Their ability to lead? Their kindness? Whatever it is, take pleasure in the fact that you too have this quality, and use them as an inspiration to develop it further.

▶ Think about one of your heroes.

▶ Write down their name on a piece of paper or in your journal.

▶ Underneath that name, write down the specific quality or qualities you admire in them.

▶ Reflect on how that quality applies to your life. How can you develop that specific quality yourself?

In this way, your hero is actually helping you to better your life, rather than making you feel inferior.

One of my heroes is Dr. Edith Eger, the psychologist and Holocaust survivor that I wrote about in my previous book. In truth, I really don't know much about Dr. Eger as a whole person. I don't know what she's like as a mother, wife, friend or colleague. But the thing I admire about her the most is her ability to choose an empowering perspective in any situation. In the midst of extreme adversity, she discovered the mental tools she needed to survive. She told me that in the Auschwitz death camp, she was able to reframe her situation so that – in her mind – she was free and it was her guards who were the prisoners. "The greatest prison you'll ever live in is the prison you create inside your mind," she told me. Edith's ability to reframe such a difficult situation has proved transformative for me. If I am ever struggling with a situation in my own life, I think about her. If she was able to reframe events in the horror of Auschwitz, I can certainly reframe them in my own life. I have used this specific quality of Edith's to inspire me, and it has genuinely changed my life for the better in more ways than I can count.

▶ **To listen to my full conversation with Dr. Edith Eger, go to Episode 253 of my *Feel Better, Live More* podcast at drchatterjee.com/253.**

VERTICAL RELATIONSHIPS

We've already discovered that our reliance on heroes can have power over us because they unconsciously take on the roles that our parents once did when we were children. But other people in life can also take on this role, not least those who sit above us in the pecking order at work. No matter how much we believe personally that all lives should be considered equal, professional relationships tend to be vertical by design. This can often lead to unhealthy reliance. After all, if we feel that our boss isn't happy with us, it's understandable that we might become stressed, anxious, depressed and reactive.

But vertical relationships can also come about outside the workplace. A few years ago, Bethany, a 45-year-old patient, came in to see me as she was struggling with fatigue, difficulty sleeping and low mood. After her blood tests came back clear, I spent some time with her trying to understand what was going on in her life. She told me that she was having problems with one of her oldest friends, Amy. They had been inseparable for more than thirty years, but Bethany had recently had some financial good fortune and was planning on opening her own Pilates studio, a long-held dream of hers. Her high-achieving friend had found this difficult and would constantly say things to undermine her new project and let Bethany know why it was destined to fail. Bethany found this really hard; I suggested that she spend some time thinking deeply about her relationship with Amy. When did their relationship start, what was going on in their lives at that time and how might the dynamics have changed over time?

She soon realized that their entire friendship had always been predicated on her being in the number two position, and almost hero-worshipping pretty and popular Amy. They had defined roles in their "friendship" that, on reflection, seemed unequal. These dynamics may have worked and served a role in the past, but they were definitely not working in the present. During one heated exchange Amy admitted that she was struggling to be happy for Bethany. It was clearly a difficult situation, but when talking to Amy about her frustrations failed to make things better, she ultimately decided she was being held back by their friendship and ended it. Healthy friendships, she realized, should be horizontal; theirs had been vertical since they were fifteen years old.

It would be easy for all the blame in this situation to fall upon Amy. But the truth is, like in almost every relationship, both people are contributing to the dynamic in one way or another. Amy enjoyed being top dog and having Bethany always do as she was asked. That may have bolstered her own self-esteem or, perhaps, helped her feel supported in a way that she hadn't felt before. On the other hand, Bethany unconsciously allowed herself to be dominated by Amy. During one consultation, she shared with me that she often felt safe and secure alongside Amy because she was able to play a supporting role to her friend, rather than be the center of attention herself, which would have made her feel uncomfortable. This dynamic helped them both in ways that they weren't even consciously aware of. And, as with all relationships, they work until they don't.

Bethany put Amy on a pedestal, like many of us do with our heroes. Whenever we do this, we create the potential for an unhealthy reliance. When that person inevitably shows their flaws, we feel disappointed and let down. But it was us who created the problem in the first place. We placed them on the pedestal. And, by doing so, we created the potential for disappointment. Had we never put them up there in the first place, we would never have felt let down. We would have accepted them as being the imperfect humans that they are.

Although it was difficult at first, within a few months, Bethany was transformed. She felt happy, content and was busy pursuing her dream of running her own Pilates studio. Her energy came back, her mood improved and her sleep problems became a thing of the past. Those complaints were never actually the real problem. They were merely a smokescreen. The real problem was her toxic relationship with her childhood friend. I'll always admire Bethany for her bravery in ending her long friendship. It must have been difficult emotionally for both the women involved. But the last time I saw her, she was thriving.

THE HERO JOURNAL

The key to ending our unhealthy reliance on external heroes and perfectionistic standards, is to redefine our definition of what a hero really is. Rather than looking outside ourselves for other people to judge ourselves against, we should focus our attention inward. If we are able to cultivate a better relationship with ourselves, practice self-compassion and work on our own self-esteem, we become much more comfortable with who we are. And, in turn, we are less likely to feel inferior to our "heroes."

One of the best ways that I know of doing this is with a simple journaling exercise:

▶ Sit in a quiet place with a notebook and note down three incidents, from the day you have just had, in which you acted like a hero.

This doesn't mean that you were as talented as your favorite musicians, sports stars or actors. It doesn't mean that you were as successful or as conventionally beautiful as some of the people you follow on social media. It definitely doesn't mean the comic book idea of a hero, which usually involves fighting evil or saving lives. What you are looking for are those small moments of heroism that we can so easily overlook in the daily stress of our lives. Did you compliment a stranger or colleague? Did you present as a positive person in a negative situation? Did you make a phone call that you have been dreading? Did you hit a deadline that was a struggle? Did

you do something difficult for your children or partner simply because you love and care for them?

This is a fantastic practice for anyone, but especially for people who struggle with issues around perfectionism. Most of us show up as a hero every day of our lives, but the problem is that we most often focus on the negatives of our behavior and forget the positives. By sending a regular positive signal to ourselves

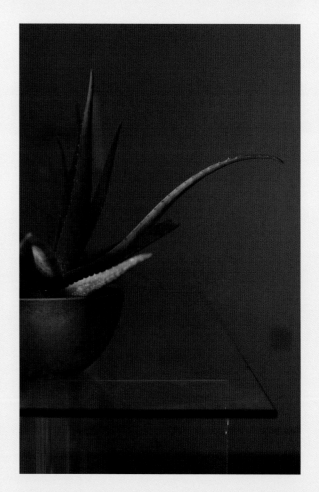

that we are heroic in our own important ways, we loosen our reliance on the external heroes whose standards are impossible to meet. We rely less on the world around us, and more on ourselves. This is the essence of Minimal Reliance, and is a wonderful basis for a life of thriving.

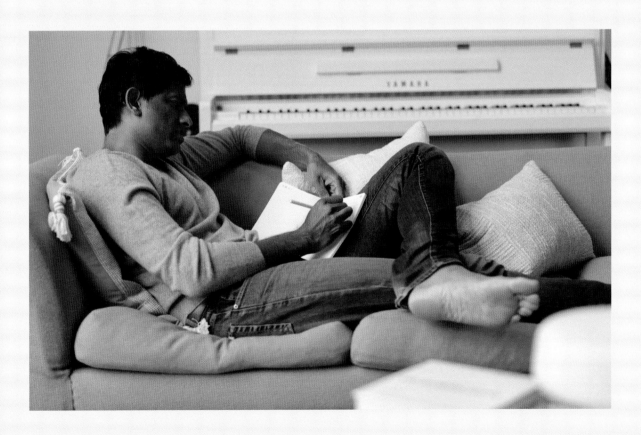

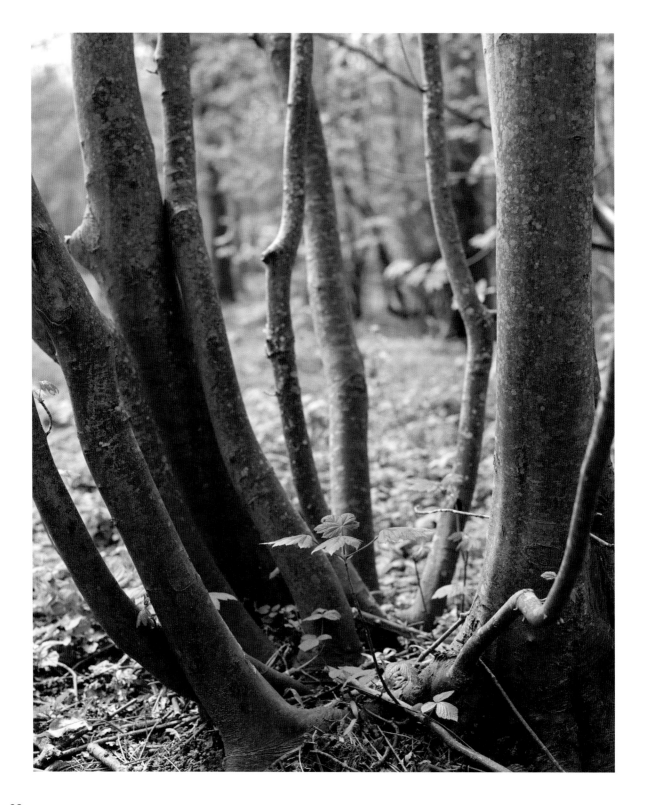

CONCLUSION

▶ We are biologically programmed to seek out heroes to mimic. This programming is designed for life in the hunter-gatherer tribe, when we would seek out and mimic wise elders. In the modern environment we are surrounded by media-created heroes who make for highly distorted models for us to copy and measure ourselves against.

▶ Because we are only shown the best moments of these modern heroes' lives, and because they appear to be exceptional in terms of their talent and beauty standards, our subconscious minds are given an unrealistic and impossible bar to reach. This has led to an epidemic of perfectionism, in which many of us feel like failures because we simply don't measure up.

▶ We can also make heroes of the people we share our lives with. When we do this, our relationships can easily become unhealthily "vertical," with us in a subordinate position that can undermine our self-esteem and our ability to grow.

▶ It's important that we choose our heroes intentionally. Rather than leaving it to our subconscious minds to pick out people to idolize and copy, we can mindfully decide what a "hero" is to us, and choose who we would like to be inspired by in the way that we live our lives.

▶ By redefining our heroes, we avoid the psychological pitfall of perfectionism, which can all too easily make us feel that we're not good enough. This can lead to anxiety, depression and mood disorders and can put the body in a damaging stress state, making us more susceptible to a wide variety of physical illnesses. It will also make it much more likely that we'll comfort ourselves with unhealthy habits.

3. BE YOURSELF

Reliance on being liked

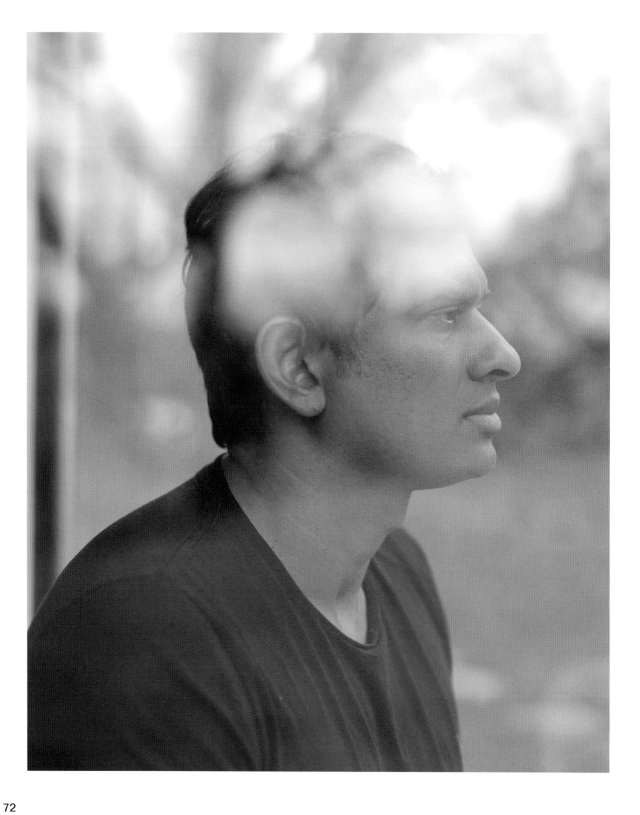

Let me tell you about one of the most significant days of my life, a day that would profoundly change who I was for more than a decade. I was fourteen years old and a student at Manchester Grammar School. The bell had just rung for the lunch break and I ran excitedly on to the playing fields to join my friends, who were all standing together in a group of six. When I reached them and tried to join in, they all looked at each other, smirking as if sharing some private joke, and walked off without me. Their rejection came out of nowhere and felt utterly brutal. I spent the rest of that lunch hour alone and in tears.

Over the next few days, I invested a lot of energy trying to find another group to fit in with. I quickly realized that finding a new set of friends would mean changing who I was – observing what kinds of people were in what kinds of groups and morphing so I fitted in. So that's what I did. I became a human shape-shifter, always prepared to be whoever anyone wanted me to be, just so they wouldn't reject me.

All throughout my teens, and right through my twenties, that was who I was. I became the guy who never wanted to be any trouble to anyone. I was the guy who would reply "I don't mind" when someone asked what bar we should go to. I was the guy who would say "you choose" when we were deciding which restaurant to eat in and so would end up eating food I didn't like while pretending I loved it. My whole modus operandi for getting on in life could be summed up as, "I'm not going to make a fuss. I'm going to fit in." But all this came at a massive emotional cost. Something inside me would rebel against the people-pleaser I had become. I'd get frustrated but I'd never show my frustration, because that would risk someone not liking me.

When I started dating Vidh, people-pleasing became a problem I could no longer ignore. After we met, I thought the way to make her like me was to give her everything she wanted. When we'd go out on restaurant dates and she couldn't decide between two dishes, I'd say, "order them both and I'll have the one that you don't want." To my surprise and confusion, this kind of behavior began to frustrate her. It turned out that Vidh didn't want me to simply please her by saying all the "right" things. She wanted a man who knew his own mind. But I couldn't understand what I was doing wrong. I was so habituated into the process of changing who I was to avoid rejection from other people, I wasn't even conscious I was doing it.

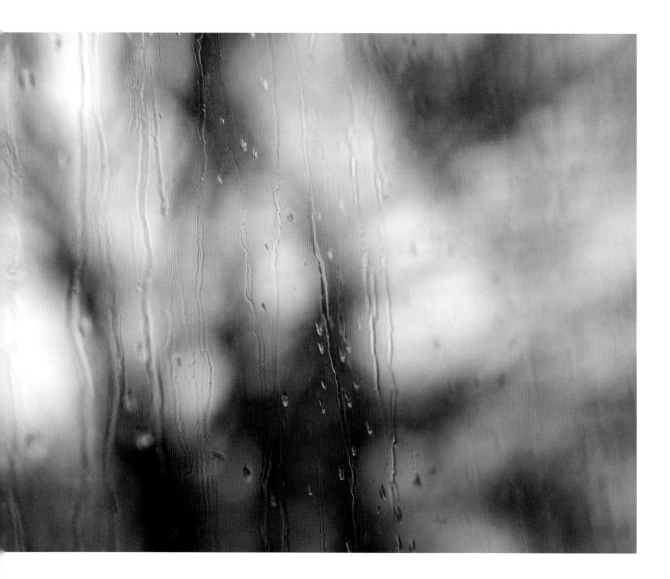

ONLY YOU CAN JUDGE YOU

It took a lot of work to process the social rejection I suffered at the formative age of fourteen. It involved a lot of heartache, self-reflection and a type of therapy called Internal Family Systems. But it was absolutely worth it. It's simply not possible to thrive if you're *overly* dependent on the approval of other people. It's crucial that we're able to look at ourselves in the mirror, before we go to bed, and say: "I'm OK with who I was today." At the end of the day, *we* should be our own ultimate judge, not other people.

Validation-seeking is both hugely common and hugely damaging. If we continually rely on other people's assessments of us to feel good, we will never feel free. Ultimately if someone doesn't like us or disagrees with something we said or did, it's out of our control. We don't have the power to climb inside their minds and change them. What we can control are our actions and values. It's inevitable that we will meet people in life who don't agree with the things we do and believe, and this will undoubtedly cause a bit of social friction, which may feel uncomfortable. It might be that these people don't like us because there's a genuine clash of values. But I'd argue that, if you do have the courage to stop people-pleasing, it's likely that one of the reasons they're pushing back is because they feel threatened by this new, improved and more assertive you.

Think of the most charismatic individuals you've encountered. Did they bend and twist themselves, changing who they were to match the people around them? Or were they happy and content just being themselves. Some of the most impressive people I know are very much the latter. They have the kind of confidence that comes with truly knowing who they are, accepting who they are, and feeling positive about taking who they are into any social situation. Of course, this doesn't mean that everyone is going to like them and agree with what they are saying. But because they are minimally reliant on validation from others, they are completely OK with this and don't allow it to change who they are.

THE GIFT OF YOURSELF

Minimally reliant people are like magnets. Others just want to be around them. Why? A part of the reason is that, subconsciously, they know they'll benefit somehow from being close to them. Relationships between minimally reliant people, whether they're romantic, professional or between friends, are generative: they generate positive benefits for everyone inside them. When we're with people whose company we thrive on, they make us laugh, they fascinate us, they support us and surprise us. Relationships like these are only possible when we're generous enough to truly be who we are. When we're in people-pleasing mode, we selfishly withhold the gift of ourselves, and this means everyone in the relationship loses.

And it's honestly true that you are a gift. Despite how this might sound, accepting that you're a gift isn't in any way narcissistic. It's not saying that you're better than anyone else. The fact is, everyone's a gift. We all have different personalities, different perspectives and different life experiences. These are the gifts we can bring to our friends, lovers, colleagues and family members. When we hold important parts of ourselves back, we make it impossible for the people around us to really know us. As my friend Dr. Gabor Maté, the trauma expert and author of *The Myth of Normal,* so eloquently puts it, "If you want to be liked, just please everybody. Never say no. Take everything on. Be responsible for how other people feel. Never disappoint anybody. They're all gonna like you. But nobody's gonna love you, because they don't know you."

To be clear, there's obviously nothing wrong with being there for other people. And sometimes putting yourself out when the occasion demands is the right thing to do. But if doing things for others at the expense of yourself is your default way of being, as it is for many, the consequences for your physical and mental health can be severe. People-pleasing is tiring and exhausting. It can lead to burnout, chronically overextending yourself and a lot of internal rage. It can also impact your sleep and the quality of your close relationships. As the pioneering endocrinologist Hans Selye writes: "The biggest stresses in human beings are emotional ones. The biggest stressor of all is trying to be who you're not."

When we're not being our true selves with others, due to a fear of not being liked, we risk being driven to depression, anxiety and low self-esteem. And, because we are not living authentically, we generate a huge amount of internal pain, which we

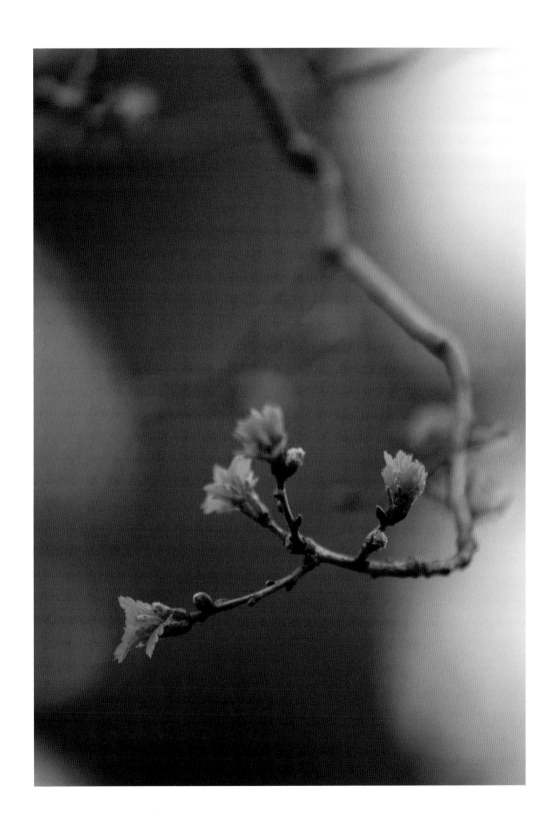

unsuccessfully try to soothe with unhealthy behaviors, like excess sugar and alcohol consumption, which only makes things worse.

THE RESPECT BALANCE

But we should not ignore the danger here. By acknowledging that we are a gift, and that we shouldn't rely on social approval, we risk tipping into selfish and uncaring states of being. This is why it's critical to always remember that we're never pursuing zero reliance. Not caring what other people think of us at all is a recipe for disaster. Nobody will want to have anything to do with us if we end up trying to dominate others with our new, unleashed, obnoxious personality. In an ideal world everyone in our relationships will be able to bring the gift of themselves and have the space to be who they are without fear of rejection. Managing this means that all involved should consciously practice the delicate art of respect.

Respect can be a difficult, even dangerous, concept. Many people are overly dependent on receiving "respect" from other people and can easily become upset, angry and perhaps even violent towards them when they perceive they've failed to get it. We typically think of people who have big egos as being super-confident, but the truth is they're super-reliant. They may look happy and on top of the world when we meet them, but if you watch them closely, you'll notice they're watching everyone else closely, to make sure they're receiving the attention and respect they believe they're due. These people are absolutely not thriving. Their wellbeing is utterly dependent on other people; people who, ironically, they often consider to be socially beneath them.

When we're minimally reliant, we're actually looking for a healthy balance of respect. We need to respect ourselves enough to actually be ourselves and, at the same time, be respectful of others by fully accepting who they are.

CHILDHOOD ROOTS

For the vast majority of us, a chronic reliance on being liked is rooted in childhood. If we are loved unconditionally as infants, it's highly unlikely we will grow up to be people-pleasers. Being loved unconditionally – literally "without conditions" – means

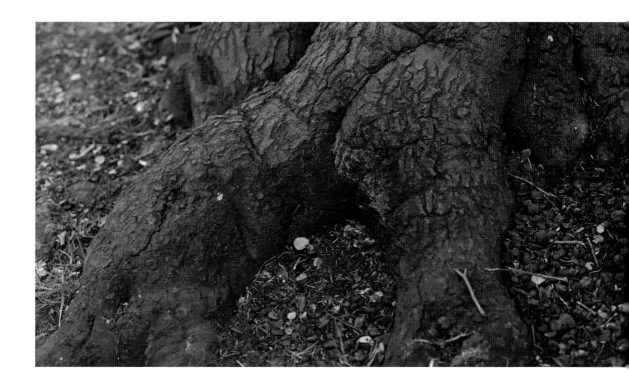

that we don't have to work to be loved and accepted. It means that we don't have be to intelligent, pretty, calm or interested in what our parents like for them to love us. It means that we will still be loved when we're angry, frustrated, sad and struggling. Of course, many of us didn't always feel this way during our childhoods, despite our parents' or primary caregivers' best efforts.

My parents did their best. They came to the UK as immigrants and faced a lot of struggle and discrimination when they got here. They heavily prioritized academic success for my brother and me, as they felt that this was the best way for us to thrive and not experience the same problems that they did. They pushed me hard but unfortunately I interpreted that as a signal that I was not fully loved for who I was. In my mind, love only came if I got certain grades or awards. This is not about blame; I know they were doing their best for me. Every situation in life has multiple interpretations. From their perspective, they were pushing me to be the best that I could be in order to thrive in life but from my perspective, as a young child, I felt that just being me was not good enough. I had to work to receive love and validation. And my interpretation had consequences for many years to come.

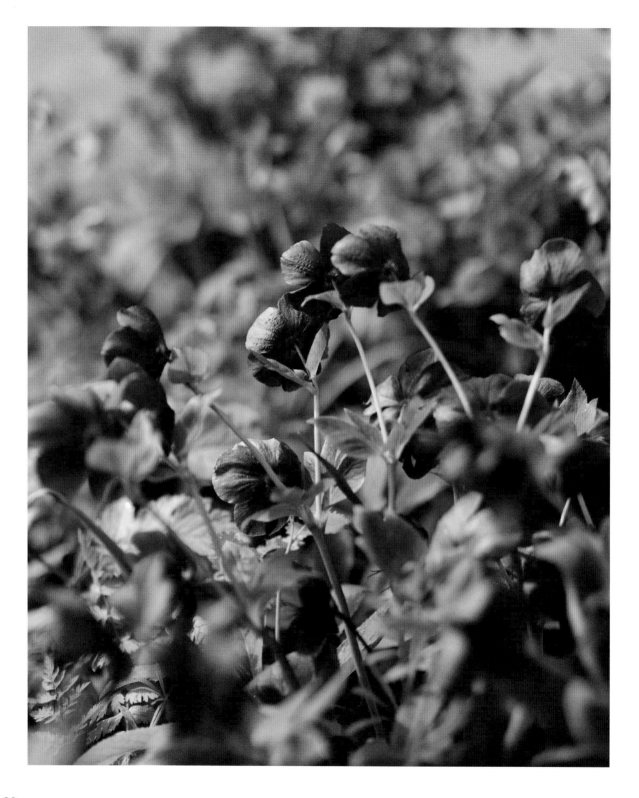

When a child is not loved unconditionally, they are forced to choose between authenticity and attachment. Faced with this choice, attachment will win every time. Love is a primal need, and children will do whatever is necessary to get it. Human infants are the weakest and most reliant animals in nature – a foal can come out of the womb, stand and start to walk within minutes, whereas humans are maximally reliant for more than a decade. In adolescence, as part of our transition into adulthood, we're supposed to learn to healthily break our childhood reliances. But we can only fully do this if we're raised in an environment in which we reliably experience unconditional love.

Strong and secure attachments formed in early childhood buffer the child from stresses later in life. The psychiatrist Dan Siegel argues that children who form secure attachments when they're young grow up to be flexible, insightful and vital. They become adults who lead happier and more fulfilled lives. He teaches that these secure bonds are formed when parents (or caregivers) provide their children with the four S's: Safe, Seen, Soothe and Secure. Of those four, he regards secure attachment as the most important. Secure attachment occurs naturally as a consequence of the first three S's being properly attended to. As Dan says, "We give our kids a secure base when we show them that they are safe, that there's someone who sees them and cares for them intimately, and that we will soothe them in distress. They then learn to keep themselves safe, to see themselves as worthy and to soothe themselves when things go wrong."

It's for reasons like these that studies show adults with stable, loving childhoods are less likely to suffer from PTSD when exposed to the same traumatic event compared to adults who did not. Even my own experience on the school playing field at the age of fourteen would in all likelihood not have bothered me as much if I had felt more secure in myself. I know from intentionally excavating my past that the core issue of not feeling good enough in who I was started long before my teenage years. I can now see that, even at the age of five or six, there were experiences that I interpreted as me not being good enough unless I performed and changed who I was. On top of that, it is no surprise that the abandonment I felt at school at the age of fourteen affected me so much. It reinforced my existing conditioning.

▶ **You can listen to each of the four wonderful conversations I've had with Dr. Gabor Maté on my podcast by going to drchatterjee.com/gabor.**

CASE STUDY

Amanda came to see me with a painful wrist. As I was examining it, as tenderly as I could, I naturally asked how she'd injured herself. "I knew you were going to ask me that," she said, with an irritable sigh.

"You don't have to tell me if you don't want," I smiled at her. "But we do need to get it sorted."

"Thanks," she said. And then, after a long silence. "Well, I punched a wall, if you must know."

To my surprise, I could see that Amanda was struggling not to cry. "It's so ridiculous," she said. "I don't know what's wrong with me. It was so utterly stupid. I was cross with my mother about the dog walker. Or the lack of a flippin' dog walker, to be precise."

Amanda explained that her mum had been struggling to walk her three dogs since her husband, Amanda's dad, had died six months earlier because her mobility issues had gotten worse. "She's constantly asking me to do it. Don't get me wrong, I love her dogs. I love them very much, I really do. But she's forty-five minutes away. So it's nearly three hours, all in. And she's got me going round there, I don't know, two or three times a week? There's no reason she can't get a dog walker. No reason whatsoever. If she's comfortable enough to get her shop from Ocado, she's comfortable enough to get a dog walker, that's what I say. I don't know when she got so selfish. She wasn't like this before Dad died. It's absolutely infuriating."

When I asked Amanda if she'd spoken to her mum about her feelings, she shook her head. "I get what you're saying, but I couldn't. I'm an only child, I'm all she's got. It would break her heart to think I wouldn't be there for her. I couldn't do it to her. So I just need to get on with it. Suck it up."

"But you're obviously very stressed about this," I said. "You've damaged your wrist. I'm wondering what else might be getting damaged?"

"It does interfere with things," she admitted. "I have two teenage daughters that need ferrying around. My husband works late. He's noticed it's affecting me. And, if I'm perfectly honest, it's affecting my marriage as well."

"Look, we'll check up on your wrist in a couple of weeks," I said. "In the meantime, I really think that you should talk to your mum. I would recommend that you speak to her when you are feeling calm and unrushed. And, remember, you don't actually know what is going on inside her head, so don't throw any accusations at her. Just try your best to tell her how you feel, when she asks you to walk the dogs."

Two weeks later, it was immediately clear that it wasn't just Amanda's wrist that had made a dramatic recovery. Gone was the slightly defensive and frustrated person I'd seen a fortnight earlier. In her place, was someone who seemed cheerful, charming and refreshed.

"Well, it was a revelation," she said, grinning. "It turns out she thought that I wanted to walk the dogs. She thought she was doing me a favor, not the other way around! I couldn't believe it. She was mortified when I told her how stressed I'd been getting about it all. It was nothing to do with her being selfish. I do love her dogs. I'm so fond of them, really. But it's been decades since Mum had a busy adult life herself and I think she's forgotten what it's like not to have a spare moment. I feel terrible, to be honest. There I was telling myself all sorts of negative stories about my mother being selfish, and so on. She's got herself a walker now. I still go around when I can, but only when I choose to and have enough time."

In itself, Amanda's story was not remarkable. I've had countless patients just like her, who have allowed a reliance on being liked and accepted at all times to damage their mental and physical health. The reason she sticks in my memory is what she said about "negative stories." Because this is what we do, when we become a people-pleaser. We become resentful. And when we become resentful, our thoughts can so easily become toxic. Our mind makes our own inability to communicate, someone else's problem. We blame them for the bad feelings they cause us, when really it's our own inability to communicate and express our own needs that's the real issue.

HOW TO HAVE HEALTHY CONFLICT

When it comes to managing conflict in my marriage, one of the most helpful tools I've learned to use is building an awareness of how much mind-reading takes place between people. This is a concept I first learned about from the relationship experts Carole Robin and David Bradford when they first appeared on my podcast.

Imagine that your partner has been complaining about always having to pick your socks up from the bedroom floor. This is a perfectly reasonable complaint, not to mention a common one. But how does this sometimes play out? Your partner may start off by saying something like, "You always leave your socks on the floor and I am sick of picking them up. You just don't care about me, do you!"

Because your partner has made assumptions and jumped to conclusions about what you leaving your socks on the floor means, you may start to feel attacked and become defensive. You, perhaps, might respond angrily with, "Well, you leave your dirty mugs in the living room all the time and I spend ages picking them up and cleaning them in the kitchen. It's clear that you don't care about me." This can rapidly escalate and lead to conflict.

The main problem here is one of what I call mind-reading. Your partner cannot possibly know what's going on in your head when you were not picking your socks up. All they know

is that your socks have been left on the floor. They do not know why you left them on the floor. They also do not know that your leaving them on the floor means that "you don't care about them." When we try to project and "read the minds" of others, potentially jumping to incorrect conclusions, what usually happens is that the other party becomes defensive.

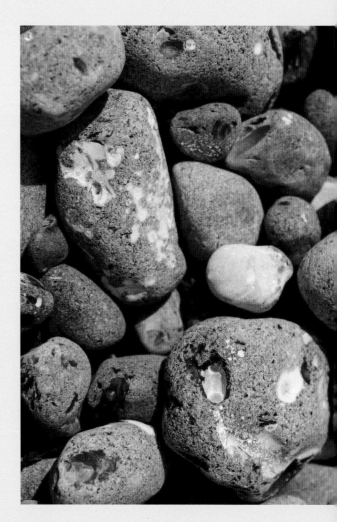

The key to productive conflict is to stick to the facts and to stick to your reality about the situation. Only you know your own reality, and only your partner knows their reality. The reason that mind-reading creates conflict is that it's often the very worst interpretation of the situation – and it's usually wrong.

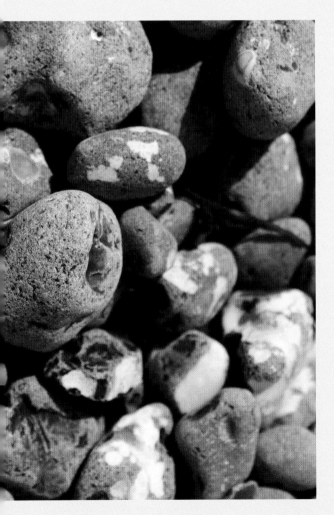

If you are the one who is frustrated about the socks, the first question to ask yourself is "Am I feeling calm at the moment?" If not, you really need to consider if this is the best time to engage. More often than not, it is better to wait until you feel grounded and more able to have a calm, non-triggered conversation. When you feel calmer, the best approach would be to say, "When you leave your socks on the floor, I feel that you don't care about me." This statement is far less likely to make a disagreement explode into conflict, because it doesn't involve mind-reading. This is your own reality. No one can argue with that. And, by sharing your reality, you are much less likely to make the other person defensive.

Whenever I'm having a difficult conversation with Vidh or my work colleagues or frankly anyone, I always make sure that I'm not making unfair assumptions or jumping to conclusions about what's going on in their heads. This leads to much healthier conflicts, and solutions.

▶ **You can listen to the wonderful conversation I had with Carole Robin and David Bradford about building exceptional relationships on Episode 177 of my *Feel Better, Live More* podcast at drchatterjee.com/177.**

BUILDING BETTER BOUNDARIES

If people-pleasing is the problem, the solution is boundaries. A boundary is something that demarcates a border. In a house, a door is a boundary. We only allow people we trust to cross it. We don't allow just anyone to come and go as they wish. This is a healthy boundary. Other forms of boundaries are those that we erect in our social lives, and can take the form of emotional boundaries, physical boundaries, material boundaries or time boundaries. Emotional boundaries might be to do with topics we don't wish to discuss in certain settings. For example, our personal life or finances might be something we don't want our partner to talk about with work colleagues or parents. Physical boundaries are to do with what constitutes appropriate physical contact. Material boundaries relate to what constitutes an appropriate use of our possessions and belongings and time boundaries relate to when we choose to give ourselves to others.

Over the past few years, I've realized that everything in my life is better when I get enough sleep. I usually go to bed at 9 p.m. and wake up at 5 a.m. In order to create the conditions around me that support this aspiration, I have had to educate my wider family about this. I have had to let them know that, unless something is truly urgent, I don't want to talk about it after 7:30 p.m. After this time, I don't want to talk about finances, house repairs or work as I'm keen to protect my "winding down" time before my 9 p.m. bedtime. It caused a little bit of tension initially as it was a change to the previous norm. But, over time, it gradually became accepted and respected. Now, it is just the way it is. The new normal.

Our relationships with others can only be truly healthy and authentic when each person understands their own boundaries, expresses them clearly, and enters a respectful negotiation with others. This is particularly important when we think about our values. Being clear on our values and expressing them to others is a kind of "value" boundary.

When I met Vidh, in my late twenties, a lot of my friends were getting married. As a result, I was deep into the "season" of bachelor parties. Thirty years ago or so, these events might have involved a boozy night in the local pub and perhaps an indulgent meal. But by the time my friends started having them, it was not unusual for a bachelor party to be a four-day weekend abroad in somewhere like Prague, Budapest or Tallinn. Vidh shared with me that she thought it inappropriate for me to go to

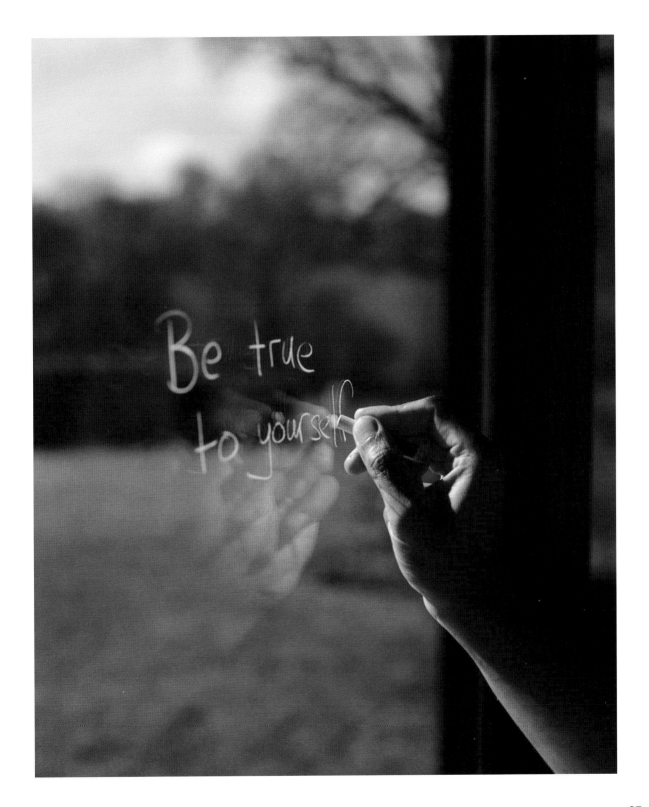

some of these bachelor parties. She felt that they were "over the top" and that it was entirely possible to celebrate my friend's wedding with the guys in a different way. To be clear, she did not have any issue with me going away and spending time with my close friends. And, she never once said that I could not go to these bachelor parties. But she was completely honest about how she felt. Initially, I was frustrated, telling her that this is what "everyone does." I felt she didn't understand, so I did attend my friends' bachelor parties, but fully aware of my wife's concerns.

Reflecting on this now, many years on, I completely see where she was coming from. She didn't feel that, now that I was married, it was appropriate for me to get boozed up, go out clubbing until the early hours and whatever else. It wasn't a case

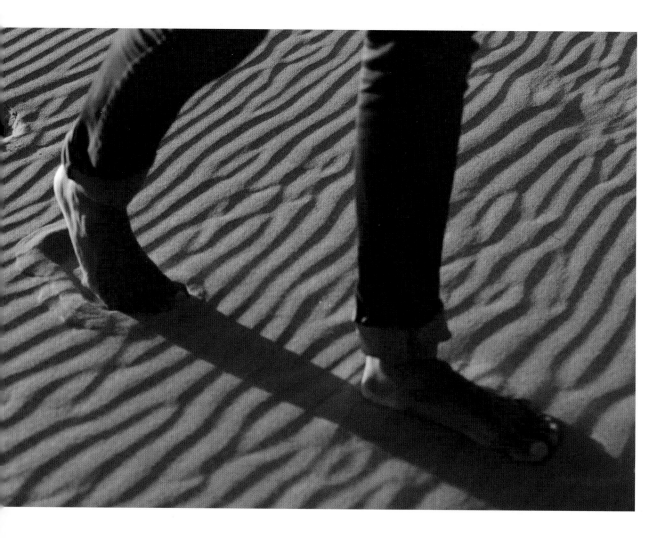

of trust. Not at all. She simply felt that, as a married man, putting myself in these situations was inappropriate. And, she had no issue calmly communicating that "value" boundary to me.

One of the reasons I found the situation so challenging back then is because I did not know what a healthy boundary really was. I don't think I even knew what the word meant in that context. Not only did I not want to let my friends down but, also, because I was unable to express my boundaries, I felt threatened by my wife expressing hers. I'm glad that Vidh felt secure enough in herself, and secure enough in our relationship, to express her own boundary. Of course, all we can ever do is express our view. We cannot make other people agree with it. We don't want to be "reliant" on people agreeing with us before we express our opinion. But I think being able to express your viewpoint is critically important for any healthy relationship, otherwise, you are not really being honest.

The consequence of not expressing your own viewpoint is that you allow and sanction things to go on as they are. You end up merely tolerating certain behaviors and then wonder why you suddenly blow up, often over something completely unrelated. By never communicating your own boundary, you allow resentment to build up inside you and that resentment flows around your body like acid. Then, when the conditions are right, maybe after a bad night's sleep, a stressful day at work, a tough commute – basically, anything that pushes you over your own personal stress threshold – that resentment and frustration spills over into a full-blown explosion. The last thing that happened was very rarely the cause. The socks being left on the floor was not actually the cause of the argument. The real cause is that you never expressed your personal boundaries in the first place.

I have come to believe that many of us abandon our own boundaries to fit in with what we think our boundaries "should" be. In countries like the UK, drinking alcohol is part and package of what you do in social situations. It's how we celebrate good times, commiserate bad times and it's an accepted lubricant for social bonding. I have spoken to many patients over the years who have admitted to me that they only drink alcohol because of the social pressure to do so. They had come to the realization that it negatively affects their sleep, their relationships, their focus and their productivity and many have even shared with me that they don't even enjoy it any more. Yet they continue to consume it because of societal pressures. This is completely understandable – we are a tribal, social species and we are handsomely rewarded when we fit in with those around us, receiving love, appreciation and respect. But, if the cost of fitting in with those around you is that you no longer respect yourself, is this really a price worth paying? Perhaps it was when you were younger, but is it still today?

This is not actually about whether you choose to drink alcohol or not. You are a grown adult who is more than capable of making that decision for yourself. The real issue is whether you are living in accordance with your own values or whether you're pretending to be someone you are not, in order to fit in with those around you.

People should be allowed to do whatever they want and live in accordance with their own values, as long as these values are not harming others. However, I do wonder how many of us have really spent time understanding and interrogating our values. How much of the time have we simply absorbed what we consider the mainstream narrative to be. If you want to thrive, you have to be less reliant on what you think your boundaries should be. You have to get clear on what they actually are and learn to express them. There is no right or wrong here – your values are your values. We all need to figure out what works for us. And, we all have the right to have personal boundaries that, at times, are at odds with the culture we live in. It doesn't mean that living in accordance with them will always be easy, but to live a happy and contented life, sometimes it will be necessary. It's also important that we don't fall into the trap of believing our boundaries are right for everyone else. I completely respect everyone's right to do what is important to them. But many of us are going along with mainstream narratives because we think that is how we should feel, rather than it being how we actually feel. It is your life. So make sure you are living it your way.

▶ Where in your life are you accepting things that compromise your values?

▶ Where in your life are you not clear on your values?

▶ And, where in your life are you clear on your values but have not expressed them to the people around you?

When we're unaccustomed to setting boundaries with other people, doing so can feel uncomfortable at first. We may feel that we're letting people down or upsetting them or appearing somehow unreasonable. There can even be a bit of pushback from others who are not used to us asserting our authentic self. If we've always constantly bowed to their demands, they can feel confused and frustrated. It's important not to be too harsh with these people. They're simply responding to who we used to be, not who we are in the process of becoming. If the relationship becomes deeply damaged by our putting up boundaries, perhaps this is a signal that the other person isn't yet able to put up boundaries of their own and, as a consequence, feels threatened by yours. In the short term, this may result in a bit of tension and distance but, over time, it can sometimes become a stimulus for positive change. By seeing you establish appropriate boundaries, they are inspired to be able to do the same thing for themselves. This is a fantastic outcome. It doesn't always happen this way, however, and sometimes it becomes clear that severing ties with them might actually be the best course of action.

If we are to achieve Minimal Reliance, we need to become OK with being disliked. The cost of trying to be liked by everyone is that we end up not liking ourselves. We lose touch with who we are, as we perform our life instead of living it. A lack of boundaries also invites a lack of respect from others. This makes us angry and volatile as we feel everyone else is treating us as a lesser being and pushing us around. We blame them for what's happening, instead of realizing that the root of the problem lies within us. When we discover our boundaries, we rediscover who we are. When we communicate our boundaries to others, we begin to consciously live as who we are. The angriness and blaming disappears, and we earn respect from other people – and ourselves.

"The cost of being liked by everyone is that we end up not liking ourselves."

It's not just our emotional health that improves when we communicate our boundaries, we become physically healthier too, as we are better able to look after ourselves and prioritize things like rest and sleep. But there is also another reason that our physical health may potentially improve that is often not spoken about nor considered.

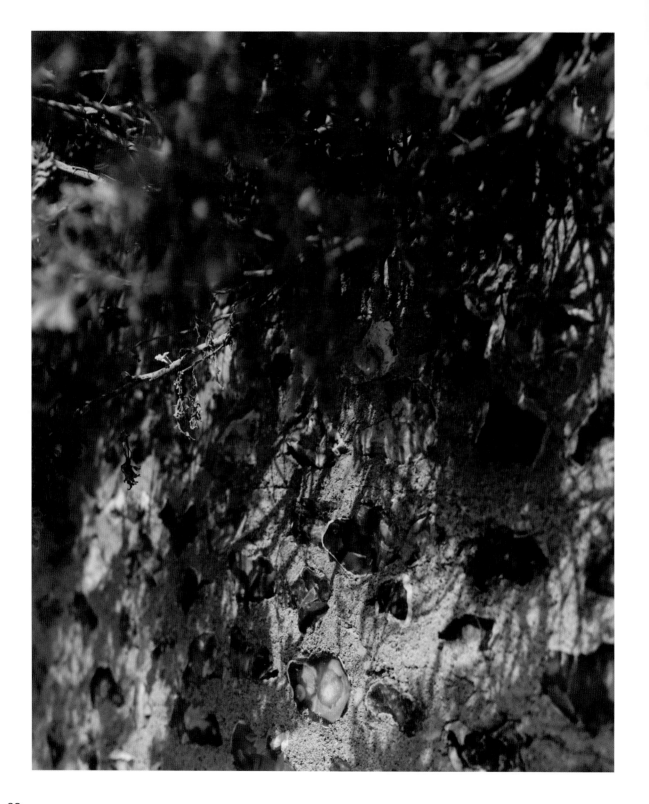

Dr. Gabor Maté has found that being overly concerned with the emotional needs of others while at the same time suppressing our own needs, is a characteristic that's present in many cases of malignancy and chronic disease. Elsewhere, there is ample research that shows a strong association between people who are unable to truly express their emotions and the presence of certain autoimmune diseases. All the way back in 1957, the astute physician Dr. C.E.G. Robinson wrote that patients with the autoimmune condition rheumatoid arthritis, "usually tried very hard to please both in professional and personal contacts, and either concealed hostility or expressed it indirectly. Many of them were perfectionistic."

While observations like these are not definitive proof that these traits directly cause the onset of these chronic diseases, they do very much reflect what I have observed myself over two decades of clinical practice. At the very least, we should be considering these emotional factors as possible contributors alongside established risk factors such as chronic stress and physical inactivity and do what we can to address them. Whenever I have shared research like this with my patients or the public, it is common for some people to become defensive. They often say, "What are you saying? That I did this to myself?" In fact, these kinds of responses are telling in and of themselves and speak to the deep insecurities that people who are excessive people-pleasers often hold. The point of my raising awareness of these observations is to empower people. It is not about blame; it is about helping people understand that the way you think and the way you interact with others influences your physical health just like the food you choose to put inside your mouth does. If you are not aware of that, you may not have the motivation to start making changes. And it's important to remember that these internal tendencies – the desire to be liked and the fear of being disliked – are usually unconscious. We think that who we are is how we have to stay. But it isn't. Who we are right now is not necessarily who we actually are. It is simply who we became. And, if we want to, we can unbecome it.

As ever, it is crucial that we don't take these principles too far. Some boundaries, such as appropriate physical contact, should never be crossed but we must be mindful that we don't allow healthy boundary-building to become an excuse for being selfish and uncooperative with others. Not all boundaries have to be rigid and impenetrable. It is much better if we allow them to be porous. If someone is truly in need, for example, you may well be prepared to make exceptions and allow certain boundaries to be crossed. In my experience, there is rarely such a thing as a "perfect" boundary that is static and holds true in every situation.

BUILDING BOUNDARIES

Building boundaries can create friction. Answering these questions will help reassure you emotionally and focus your thoughts in the right way.

► Do you ever struggle to say no?

► Ask yourself, why? What are you afraid of?

► What's the worst that will happen if you say no?

► What's the best thing that will happen if you say no?

► What's the most likely thing that will happen if you say no?

► Is someone making unreasonable demands of you? If so, understand that a boundary has been crossed and clearly communicate it with this person, when you are feeling calm.

► Is the demand arguably reasonable? If so, meditate on why it feels like a boundary for you. If you ultimately decide you still don't want to do it, explain your issues calmly and be prepared to enter a negotiation.

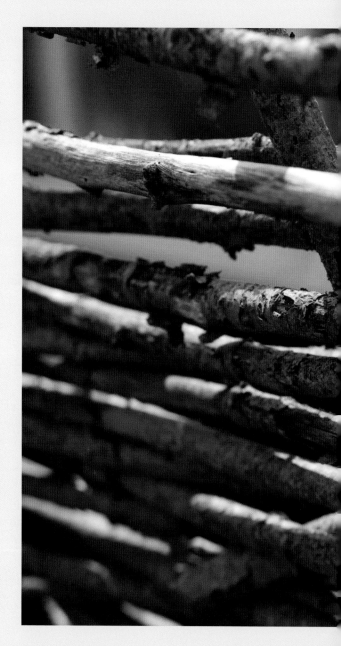

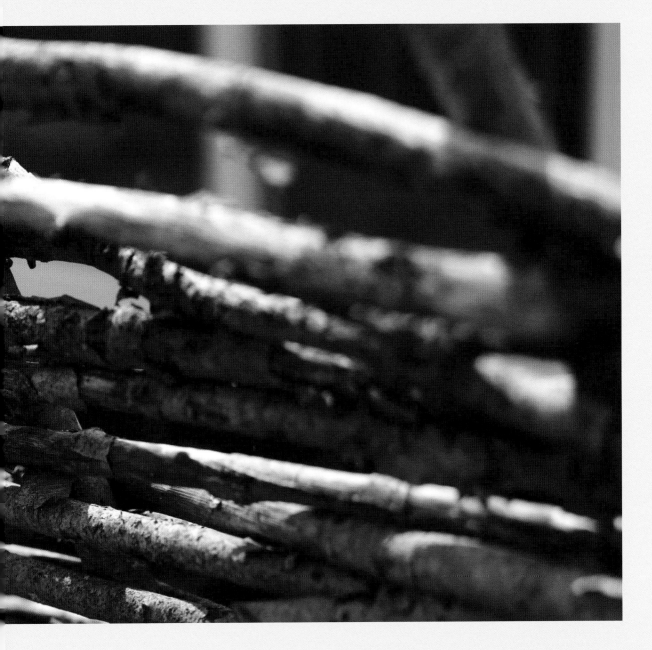

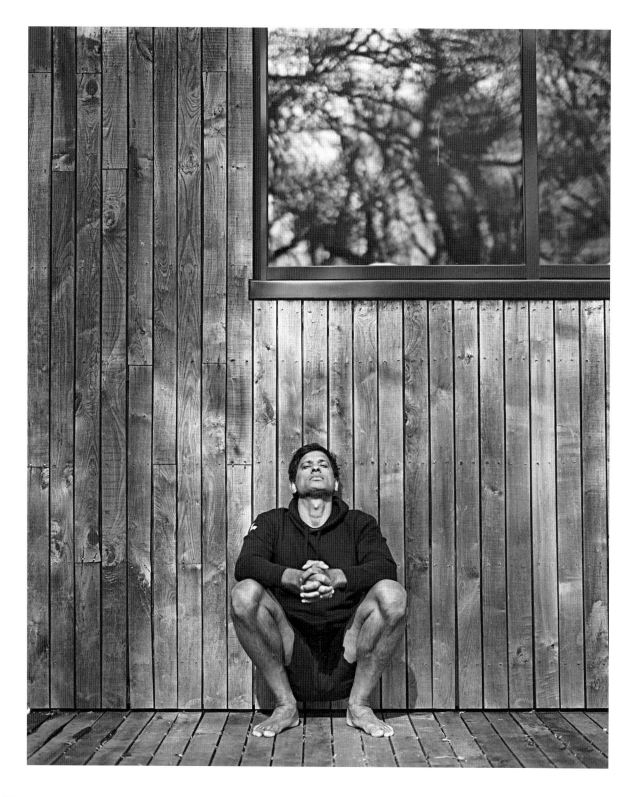

CONCLUSION

▶ Social rejection is a universal human fear. We all want to be liked. But too many of us become reliant on being liked by everyone. As a result, we become people-pleasers.

▶ When we people-please, it often feels like we're being nice and kind. After all, what could be wrong with wanting to please people? The problem is, we become massively reliant on the approval of everyone we meet. This universal approval is impossible to achieve. Additionally, we become overly subservient, hiding who we really are in an attempt to become the person someone else wants us to be. Ironically, over time, this tends to make us less lovable.

▶ We can break the reliance on being liked by learning to accept and respect who we are. Everyone is different, and this difference is our gift to other people.

▶ We should also learn to make healthy boundaries. A minimally reliant person is someone who is able to respectfully say no. We have a duty to protect our own mental health and physical health, not to mention our resources, be they in the form of time, money or energy.

▶ When we feel unable to express our emotions and subsequently suppress our own needs, we become anxious, reactive and depressed. In some cases, we may also be making ourselves more susceptible to becoming sick in the future. Breaking this reliance will have huge positive benefits for our physical health, mental health and our self-esteem.

▶ When we show our friends, partners and colleagues who we really are, they will love us for who we really are. It's only under these conditions that we can truly feel loved.

4.
EMBRACE DISCOMFORT

Reliance on comfort

Five years ago, I'd never swum in the ocean. My parents were immigrants to the UK from India, so whenever we went on vacation we would either travel back to India to see family or go sightseeing in iconic European cities. Swimming in the sea just wasn't something that families like ours, who lived a long way from the coast, did. But then I got invited to an event called SwimRun. The idea was that participants would wear a wetsuit and running shoes, run for a short while, swim for a bit in the sea, often to an island, to run for a bit before getting back in the ocean and so on. Despite my inexperience with the ocean, I was a decent enough swimmer at the pool and it sounded like fun, so I agreed to take part.

When the time for the SwimRun came around, though, I began to have second thoughts. I phoned the organizer up a few days before the event and told him I'd come along to watch, but I wouldn't take part because I hadn't done enough training. The truth is, I was nervous about swimming in the open sea and the organizer picked up on how I was feeling. He said, "Rangan, if you ever want to try this, this is the safest way. We'll have safety boats everywhere. We won't let you get in trouble." Reassured, I ordered myself a wetsuit. The next Saturday morning I found myself in Devon, pulling on the stretchy outfit for the first time, wondering if they were really meant to be so ridiculously tight.

Even before I got in the sea, I felt out of my depth. Everyone on the beach looked like pros with their special paddles and ropes and other specialist equipment. Trying to steady my nerves, I ran into the waves for my first swim, which was 250 meters – a distance I'd have no trouble completing in a pool. But even with the wetsuit on, it was freezing cold. As soon as I could no longer see the bottom, about 50 meters

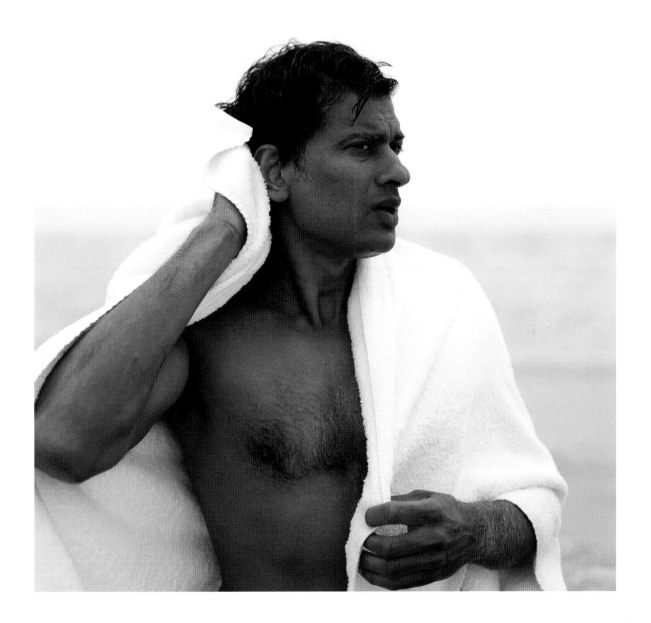

in, I began to panic. I felt really scared and my breathing became fast and shallow. I paddled frantically, trying my best to keep my chin above the water and get my nerve back. I repeatedly told myself, "Just get yourself to dry land and get out of here. You're never getting in this damn ocean again."

When I finally completed the swim and got my feet back on to terra firma, I felt slightly calmer. I decided I'd do the next, 500-meter run and then pull out. But when I reached the next bit of sea I thought, "Do you know what? Sod it. I will do this swim. Then I'll get out."

In the end, I completed the whole event. I can't tell you how incredible I felt at the end. Even though my time of one hour and forty-six minutes was far from the best, I'm sure I felt more elated than some of the pros who'd already had their lunch long before I hit the finish line. I had pushed myself well into my discomfort zone and then carried on pushing. I had conquered the noisy part of myself that wanted safety and ease. By doing so I'd achieved something that, less than two hours earlier, I'd believed was truly impossible.

Fast-forward to today and I genuinely love ocean swimming. A few months after that virgin event, I took part in another SwimRun event in France with my nine-year-old son as my partner. The day of the race was a windy and blustery day, and the waves were crashing about on the ocean. We went out for our swims, me with my son tied to my waist. Yes, it was challenging, but we navigated the entire race and completed it. Just four months beforehand, I was panicking and petrified in a shallow part of a much calmer sea; now, I was taking my nine-year-old boy out into a wavy ocean, with no concerns.

To be clear, I wasn't doing anything unsafe or risky. It was a properly managed event with lifeguards and safety boats everywhere. But the fact that I was able to complete the event and look after my son at the same time sent a very powerful signal to my brain: that I could rely on myself. As a father, it is an incredible feeling to know that I am physically capable of looking after him should things ever get tricky.

THE COST OF COMFORT

My experience at SwimRun brought into a focus how fundamentally important it is for us to be able to face life's inevitable moments of discomfort. We'll simply never be able to thrive if we're reliant on comfort and coziness at all times. For all its advantages, the modern world fools us into believing that comfort is the natural state of existence, and anything that isn't comfortable is to be rejected and complained about. Industry makes millions by figuring out new ways of making us marginally more comfortable than we used to be, often presenting us with perceived "discomforts" and then providing the solutions that they convince us will make our lives better. When I was a kid, I honestly cannot remember a single time when we went out to get takeout. Now we have delivery services bringing hot, fresh meals to our door without us even having to get off our chairs. Even our supermarket shopping is brought to our homes in specially built vans, at whatever hour we decide is most convenient for us. Of course there's nothing wrong, in isolation, with seeking comfort and convenience. The problem is we've got to a point where many of us are overdosing on it, and it's making us sick.

Most of the chronic diseases we are suffering from today can be directly linked to our reliance on comfort. Type 2 diabetes, for example, currently affects 7 million people in the UK alone. It is a condition that occurs because excess fat has accumulated inside our bodies, which damages our metabolism. This causes our blood glucose levels to rise, which results in kidney, eye, circulation and nerve problems, to name just a few. A condition like this can pretty much only exist in a world of comfort and convenience. For most of our existence, humans have had to move their bodies every day to acquire their food and cook it. It would have been almost impossible for excess fat to build up inside our bodies over a long period of time, with all the damaging effects on our health that this causes. Our bodies still expect this kind of daily effort and movement. Today, however, most of us live lives of excessive physical comfort, with our sofas, sedentary jobs, cars and home deliveries of anything you could possibly imagine, from food to books to lightbulbs. And it's killing us. Scientific research shows clearly that lack of movement is one of the leading causes of premature death globally, increasing our risk of cancer, obesity, heart attacks, strokes and type 2 diabetes.

The problem is, while we need a certain amount of movement to be healthy, the brain is programmed to conserve energy whenever and wherever possible. This is because we evolved in an environment of scarcity, in which periods of involuntary fasting would have been inevitable. The Swedish psychiatrist Anders Hansen explained on my podcast that, as well as being lazy, the brain wants us to be anxious and fat. In times when survival was front of mind, being anxious enabled us to identify danger, while putting on fat allowed us to store precious energy. Unlike us, our ancestors didn't have to seek discomfort intentionally. Life was already full of discomfort, and our minds and bodies still thrive best when we are regularly doing the kinds of things that we would have had to do in the much more hostile and difficult world that our ancestors inhabited.

Physical exercise is the intentional practice of controlled discomfort. Regularly exercising the body makes it more resilient because we are essentially putting it through manageable amounts of stress. As it works to handle the stress load we've put it under, and then returns to normal, it is "practicing" how to deal with stress. This means that when a bigger load of stress comes into our life – which it inevitably will – we'll be more ready and able to handle it. In fact, a 2021 study found that just eight weeks of aerobic exercise improved resilience and the ability to react to non-exercise stressors. In this study, participants moved their bodies just three times per week, with sessions varying from 30 to 50 minutes.

WE ARE GETTING WEAKER

Our over-reliance on comfort doesn't only affect us as adults, it affects our kids as well. A rough but useful yardstick of judging how fit we are is our ability to run. To run well means we have good cardiovascular health as well as the physical and psychological ability to endure discomfort. People who have good aerobic fitness have a significantly decreased risk of heart attacks and strokes in later life. A scientific review of fifty studies that involved 25 million children from twenty-eight countries found that today's kids take, on average, ninety seconds longer to run a mile than children did in the 1980s. This is a shocking but extremely telling finding. As we rely more and more on things outside ourselves to solve all our problems for us, the ability of our own minds and bodies to survive and thrive deteriorates.

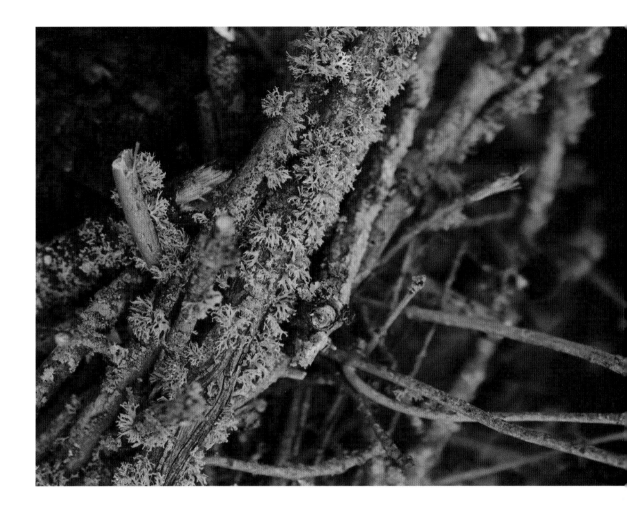

This reliance on comfort also affects our moods. When we outsource our reliance, whether that's to other people or companies and services, we become vulnerable to their failings. Just like children, when things in our external world let us down, we experience low mood and complain and often end up having an embarrassing tantrum. Not long ago I found myself on a train to London with a friend who was getting frustrated because the app that was supposed to get a bottle of water delivered to his seat wouldn't work. Because I'd been thinking so much about Minimal Reliance, I reflected on the absurdity of the situation. There we were in a warm carriage in the middle of winter, traveling at over one hundred miles an hour to one of the great capital cities of the world, and my friend's mood had been spoiled because he had to actually stand up and walk to the cafe in a different carriage to get a drink.

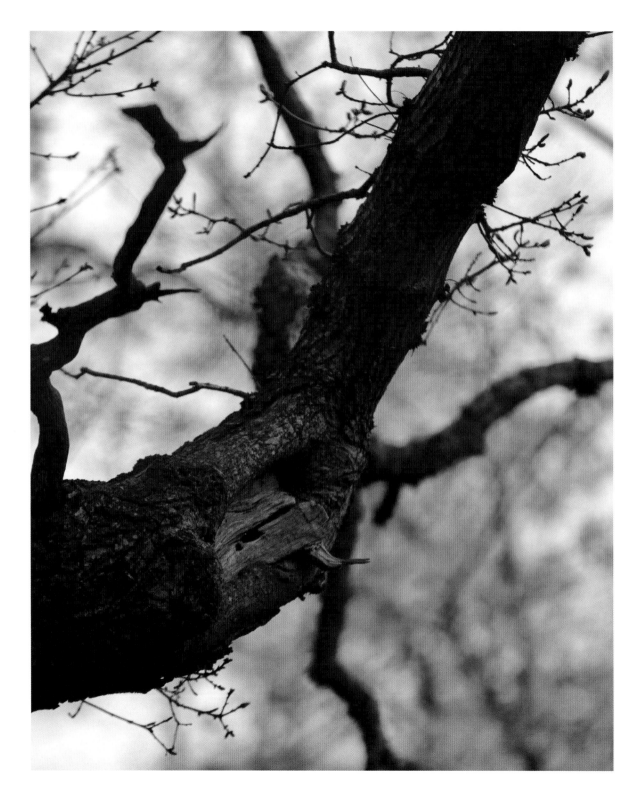

This is one of the traps of modern life. We're seduced into becoming reliant on companies and services, which (when they work) make us briefly more comfortable, while putting us in a state of permanent dependency. But no matter how hard companies and services work to remove problems from our life, we'll never stop experiencing them, no matter how easy life becomes. Evidence for this is seen in research by Harvard psychologists David Levari and Daniel Gilbert that shows that the human brain will start looking for problems even when they don't exist. Levari calls this phenomenon "prevalence-induced concept change." This basically means that, as we experience fewer problems, we start to lower our threshold for what actually constitutes a problem. The psychologists conducted a series of experiments that demonstrated this, including one in which they asked participants to identify faces that appeared threatening, which they did just fine. But as the number of threatening faces they were shown was reduced, they then started to classify ordinary faces as threatening, as well.

PRACTICING DISCOMFORT

Around 2,000 years ago, the Stoic Roman philosopher Seneca would regularly "practice" poverty. Although he was born into wealth, status and privilege, he would on occasion leave his home in simple clothes and walk the streets, surviving on just bread and water and sleeping in simple accommodation. He wanted to stare at abject poverty in the face and remind himself that he could cope. This allowed him to go through life taking important risks because he was not concerned about his ability to handle a reversal of fortune. He wanted to be minimally reliant on his money and fame and know that if they were taken away from him overnight, he would still be fine.

I believe this is why Spartan Races, Tough Mudders, Ultramarathons and wild swimming are growing in popularity. People instinctively realize that comfort is bad for us and crave the knowledge that they are resilient enough to cope with life's inevitable discomforts. Currently, my favorite discomfort practice is Breath Hold Work. I don't need to tell you that, even after a short time, holding your breath becomes extremely uncomfortable. You've got your eyes shut, you can feel the tension mounting, you can feel the urge to breathe starting to come, you can feel spasms in your tummy, which is your diaphragm expanding and contracting. Your body is literally screaming, "Open your mouth!" One of the most primal threats of all is the lack of oxygen. As far as your subconscious mind is concerned, you're looking directly at death. If you can truly learn to control your mind when it's begging you to breathe, everything else life can throw at you will feel easy in comparison.

My introduction to Breath Hold Work took the form of a four-week course with a brilliant practitioner named Erwan Le Corre. In our first session he told everyone to take a deep breath, and time how long we could hold it for. I managed one minute. Four weeks later I could last four minutes and twenty seconds. It clearly wasn't my physiology – things like my lung capacity or my body's ability to tolerate rising carbon dioxide levels – that changed in just one month to make that improvement possible. It was my mind. What this showed me was just how much of our anxiety, stress and panic is the product of our minds and not actually based on true threat. It's honestly been the best self-awareness course I've done. In that moment when you're screaming to breathe, you learn that it's not willpower that gets you through life's toughest moments, it's having absolute trust that you can rely on yourself. You can only develop this enhanced form of self-trust by actively seeking discomfort.

THE RELIANCE SIGNAL

So many of us walk around feeling weak because we haven't given ourselves enough evidence to the contrary. When we do present ourselves with this evidence, we can experience growth in all other aspects of our lives. Breath Hold Work has enabled me to cope much better with everyday moments of stress and given me greater confidence to deal with whatever life throws at me. Every time I practice, I send a signal to my brain that I am resilient in the face of crisis. I tell it that it doesn't matter that the world is fundamentally uncontrollable – as long as I'm in control of myself, and my own responses to what the world throws at me, I'll be able to navigate even the wildest of storms. Sure, I might get tossed around by life and have moments of genuine fear but, when it all dies down, I know I will always be fine.

Of course, if you don't fancy the idea of Breath Hold Work, that is completely fine. There are many different ways in which you can start embracing discomfort, a variety of which I will share with you over the upcoming pages. While a lot of these practices do have physical benefits, for me their real benefit is psychological. At its core, embracing discomfort is about changing the way we feel about ourselves. One of the reasons so many of us struggle with self-worth in the modern world is because we have become conditioned to think there will always be someone or something there to look after us. Over time, this over-reliance on things outside of ourselves becomes toxic. To feel physically and mentally well, we need to know we can rely on ourselves, especially during times of stress. Over the years, I have seen this play out with my patients. Many of them seemed to have a low-grade anxiety that was built on a foundation of fragility. On a deep level, they knew that things in their life could get worse but because they had never tested themselves, they didn't actually trust themselves to be able to handle whatever came their way.

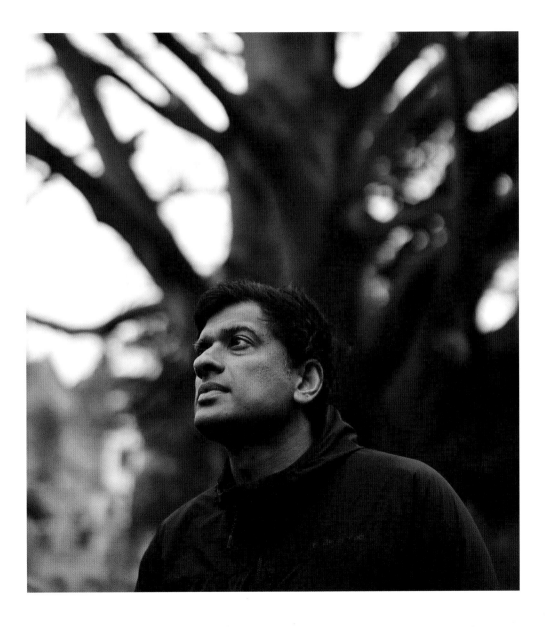

HOW TO EMBRACE DISCOMFORT

There are a variety of different ways in which we can start to embrace discomfort and give ourselves real world evidence of our own resilience. I have listed some options below, to get you thinking. As always, it's important that you choose something that appeals to you and will suit the context of your wider life. Of course, feel free to come up with your own options that are not on the list below.

RUNNING A 5K

You don't have to do a Tough Mudder or compete in the CrossFit Games to embrace discomfort. It's entirely relative to how active you are right now. If you've been relatively sedentary for a number of years, the challenge of working up towards a 5k run (or walk!) will motivate you and push you in the right direction. The simple act of getting fitter and stronger, will change the way you feel about yourself, as you will be giving yourself real-world evidence that you are a strong and adaptable human, capable of doing difficult things.

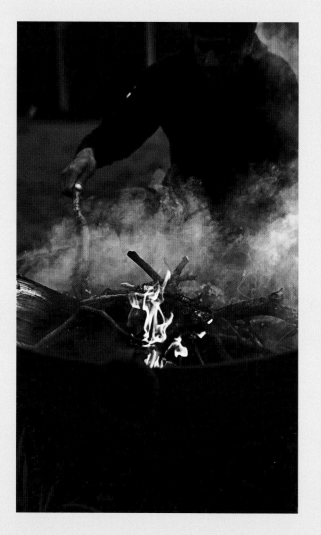

GOING OUTSIDE IN BAD WEATHER

Even going for a walk or run or bike ride in inclement weather can help you. If you are reliant on only going outside to move in good weather, what signal does that send to your brain? When you regularly exercise outside whatever the weather, you show your brain that you are a capable human being who can

COLD SHOWERS

There's growing evidence that intentionally exposing ourselves to cold temperatures – such as taking cold showers or a quick session in a cold plunge pool – can have a number of potential physiological benefits, such as increasing the amount of a type of fat in the body called brown fat, which can have beneficial effects on our metabolism. There is also emerging evidence supporting the idea that exposure to cold can be good for our immune systems. One study showed that people who take a 30-second cold shower each day at the end of their warm shower, report fewer sick days than those who don't. But, for me, their most important benefits are psychological. A short, sharp blast of cold water is like a natural steroid for the subconscious mind, boosting its resilience and its trust in itself.

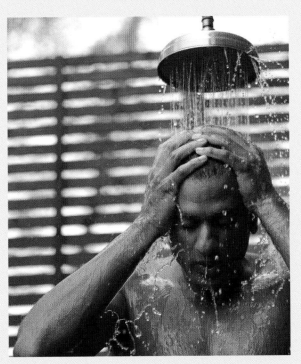

FASTING

For some people, fasting can be a transformative practice and a useful tool to tackle the diseases of comfort that are crippling healthcare systems, such as type 2 diabetes and obesity. Research has shown that it can have a variety of physical benefits. For example, it lowers levels of the hormone insulin, which can help us burn fat and increase levels of human growth hormone, which helps maintain our tissues and organs. It can also accelerate cellular repair by removing waste products from our bodies, as well as reduce levels of oxidative stress and inflammation. For me, however, just like with cold showers, the most important benefits are psychological.

In a world where many of us consume more food than our bodies need, fasting is a form of self-imposed scarcity. In my experience, it can be incredibly helpful for anyone who's ever had a problematic relationship with overconsuming things like food, alcohol, caffeine, sugar – even social media. It is a practice that teaches us that we don't have to be a slave to our cravings.

Of course, it's important to highlight that fasting may not be the most suitable practice for everyone. What is appropriate for any individual depends on their current state of health and the context of their wider lives. If, for example, you are suffering with an eating disorder or recovering from one, fasting may not be the best practice for you. At the same time, if you are carrying excess weight or your blood tests show that you are pre-diabetic, it may prove transformative.

There are various ways to fast, ranging from twelve hours without any food, to longer, multi-day fasting cycles. If this is a discomfort practice that appeals to you, I would encourage you to experiment and find out what works for you. A straightforward way to start is to make sure that you eat all of your food within a twelve-hour window each day, which means you will have twelve hours when you are fasting. This could be as simple as making sure you don't eat anything after 8 p.m. and then not eat breakfast (breaking your fast) until 8 a.m. the next morning. This is a simple practice that many people find helps them with their weight, gut health, digestion and sleep.

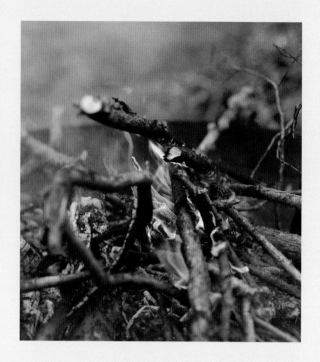

WILD CAMPING

Many people I know love the discomfort of wild camping. Wild camping is about going back to basics and getting away from most of the comforts of the modern world. Wild campers find that they become so busy with the act of just living – making shelter, keeping warm and getting food – that they simply don't have time to think about much else. Even going to the bathroom or making a coffee are activities that require a fair degree of effort.

By removing so many comforts and conveniences, they force themselves to be present. It also reminds them of who us humans really are, and how much discomfort we're able to tolerate, giving us a renewed appreciation for modern comforts like heating, comfy mattresses and sofas.

LEARNING SOMETHING NEW

Learning something new that's not easy, like a language or a musical instrument, can be incredibly beneficial, with pleasant side effects for the brain. We typically go through a huge period of learning during childhood and adolescence, but as soon as we reach our thirties, we tend to stop learning at anywhere near the same rate. Once we have found our career and feel settled, we often stop learning anything new. Too much of this kind of comfort can be problematic for our brains, and can make us more susceptible to the decline in brain function that many people experience as they get older. If languages and musical instruments are not to your taste, have a think about other activities that might appeal to you. Remember, the key is that you choose something that you find a bit difficult and challenging.

CHALLENGE YOURSELF SOCIALLY

Just as leaving our physical comfort zone makes us more physically resilient, leaving our social comfort zone makes us more socially resilient, as well.

Ways to explore discomfort socially might include volunteering at your local food bank or charity, putting in an application to join the Samaritans, or going to a local yoga class by yourself when you don't know anyone there. It could even be facing your social fears by singing or playing an instrument in public. If you are someone who feels shy and struggles to interact with strangers, you could challenge yourself to say "hello" and "how are you?" to the barista or the cashier at the supermarket.

The more you lean into this social discomfort, the more comfortable these situations become. And, as we will explore in Chapter 9, the social

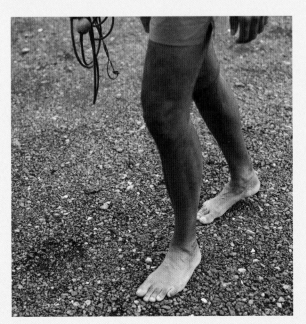

bonds we share with others are crucial for our physical and mental wellbeing.

ANNUAL CHALLENGE

Once a year, why not come up with a "big" challenge that is outside your current zone of comfort. Examples that involve physical discomfort might include a four-hour hike in nature, a 10K walk for charity, running a marathon, signing up for a SwimRun, a triathlon, an open-water swim or anything else that appeals to you. Perhaps, you have always wanted to swim but never had the opportunity to learn and now think it might be too late. Could you sign up for swimming lessons with a coach at your local pool?

More ideas to get you thinking include visiting a new country with only a backpack, sharing your art online for 100 consecutive days or taking part in a summer reading challenge. The point is to set yourself a challenge that you don't know for sure that you can do but would like to try. Although the goal is to complete it, the truth is that simply getting ready and preparing for it will teach you a lot. You will learn about your inner fears and insecurities, but you will also learn that you are capable of much more than you think, which, in turn, will grow your resilience and trust in yourself.

Note: If you are on any medication, please consult a healthcare professional before going for prolonged periods of time without food. And, if you have uncontrolled hypertension or heart disease it is not advised that you engage with cold water immersion.

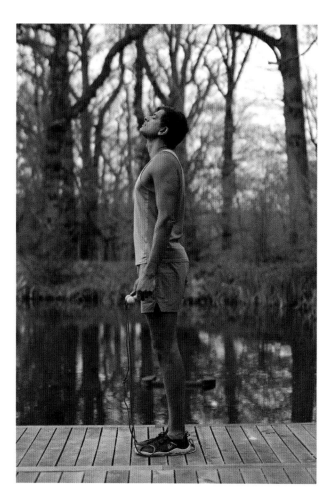

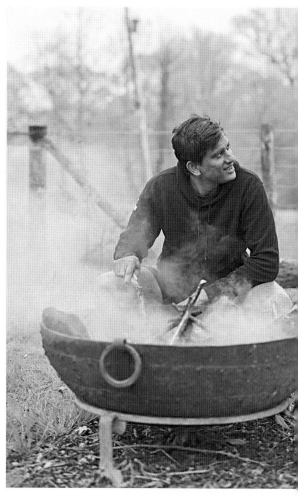

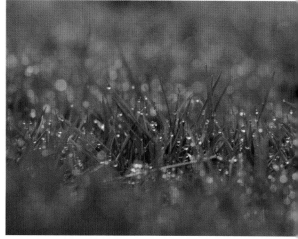

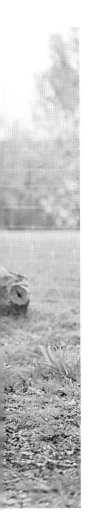

"You are capable of much
more than you think."

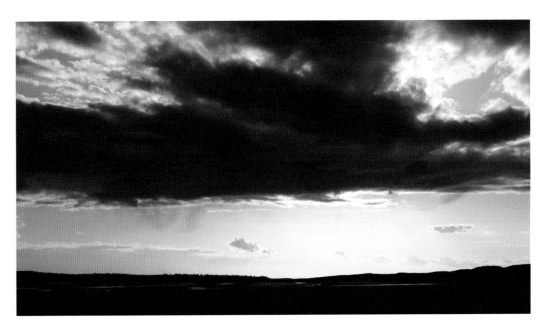

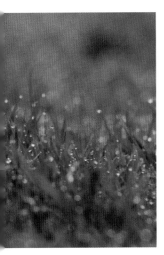

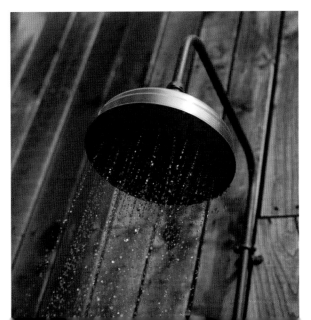

CREATE YOUR OWN
RULES FOR DISCOMFORT

Practicing discomfort doesn't always need to be a big gesture. There are many opportunities in everyday life for us to practice, with knock-on benefits for our wellbeing. Doing your meditation each morning takes more effort than drinking your coffee while scrolling Instagram, but it will help you feel calmer and in control. Turning your smartphone off one hour before bed takes more effort than watching YouTube on it, but will likely improve intimacy with your partner, as well as the quality of your sleep. Taking the stairs to get to the supermarket parking lot is harder than taking the elevator but, over time, will make you stronger and more resilient.

When you're sitting on the sofa, and the next episode of your favorite show starts playing, the easiest thing to do is to stay there. The inconvenient and uncomfortable thing to do is to stop watching, get up from the sofa and go to bed. And, of course, getting enough sleep will have a huge impact on the way you feel the following day, and improve your physical health and mental wellbeing. All of these small "uncomfortable" actions will yield incredible benefits when done consistently. However, in order to counteract our natural tendency to take the easy option, we need a strategy.

In his book *Clear Thinking*, Shane Parrish writes about replacing decisions with rules. "In a quirk of psychology, people typically don't argue with personal rules," he writes. "It turns out that rules can help us automate our

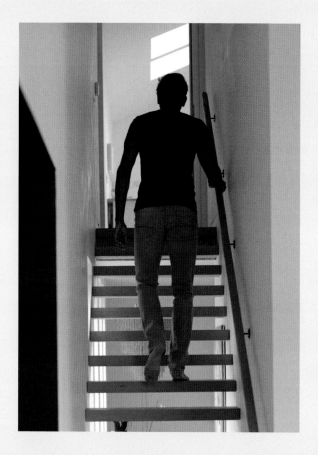

behavior to put us in a position to achieve success and accomplish our goals." The basic idea is to get away from constant decision-making, which is tiring and open to sabotage by our moment-by-moment feelings.

To help you make practicing discomfort your default mode of being, have a think about some "discomfort rules" that you can bring into your own life. Here are some simple examples to get you thinking, but feel free to come up with your own:

▶ **Always take the stairs** – so that elevators and escalators become the exception rather than the norm.

▶ **Never eat after 7 p.m.** – or at a time that suits you better. Many of our poor food choices tend to come in the evening. This one-time rule automatically eliminates them.

▶ **Never snack** – only eat at mealtimes.

▶ **Always go to parkrun** – make a commitment that every Saturday morning you are going to show up, rain or shine.

▶ **Do 30 minutes of daily movement** – it doesn't have to be anything fancy or going to a gym, just make a commitment to yourself that thirty minutes of movement every day is what you are going to do.

▶ **Never say yes to a request on the phone** – this will help reduce the likelihood of over-committing. Always say you'll have a think about it, decide and get back to the other person. If you want, you can even explain that you never say yes to requests over the phone.

▶ **Never eat a dessert alone** – this helps avoid comfort and emotional eating and means that if you do choose to eat a dessert, you can do so in the company of others, rather than to soothe loneliness.

▶ **Turn off your smartphone one hour before bed** – or at a specific time that works for you every evening. This one-time decision will have multiple downstream benefits, like enhanced sleep, more time for intimacy and a feeling of calm.

▶ **On weekdays, never start a new episode after 9 p.m.** – it is tempting to binge-watch your favorite box sets but this one-time rule will help you prevent late nights during the week. You could also have a rule that you will only ever watch one episode on week days, no matter how tempting it is to watch a second.

▶ **When you wake up, do one five-minute action for your health** – make it a promise and stick to it. This could be journaling, breathwork, meditation or a quick workout, whatever appeals to you. By keeping this promise you send your brain a signal that you are trustworthy and reliable. Doing this first thing in the morning also has an additional benefit. It becomes a little ritual that gives you a sense of order and control in a world full of chaos and uncertainty.

FOR GREATER COMFORT, CHOOSE DISCOMFORT

It's a simple fact of human existence that whatever we repeat, we get good at. The brain and body form around our habits. Most of us spend a large chunk of every day "training" ourselves for comfort; as a result, we have become excellent at it. I'm not asking you to stop enjoying life's little comforts and luxuries. This is simply about balancing them out with regular, intentional moments of discomfort. It takes a bit of discipline to do these every day, but you should see them as a workout in the gym of Minimal Reliance. Every time you practice discomfort, you become more resilient, and send your brain critical signals that you are in control and that you are capable. And in my experience, the beauty of this is that when you train for discomfort, you actually get to enjoy your comfort more. Not being reliant all the time on luxuries and conveniences allows us to indulge in them in a state of simple, pure carefreeness that we just don't experience when we're dependent on them. When we thrive, we have the freedom to choose to enjoy life's pleasures – or not.

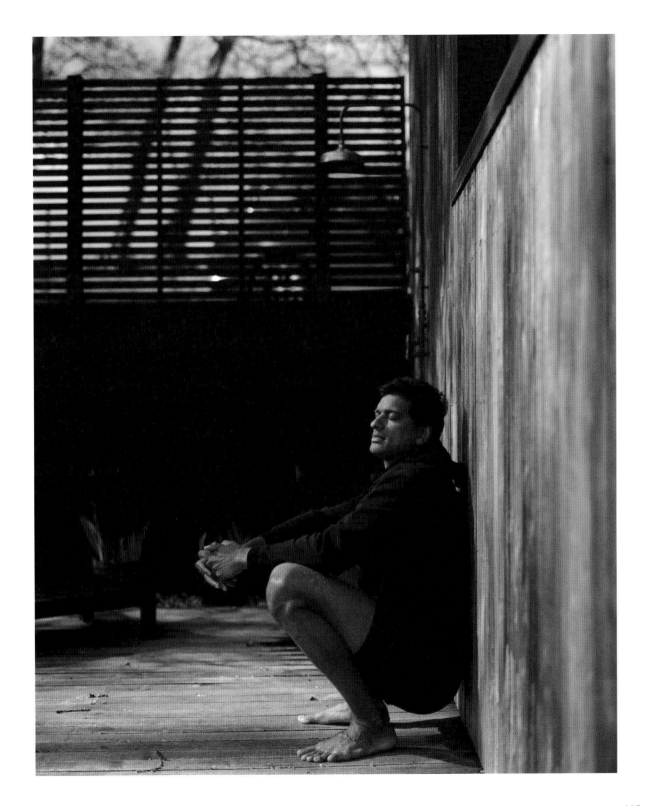

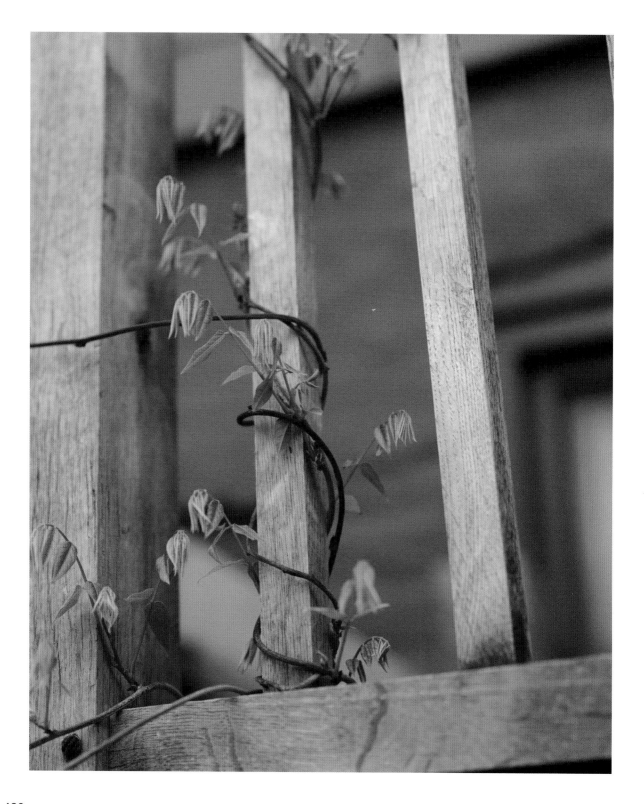

CONCLUSION

▶ Over the last 200 years, life has become immeasurably safer for people across the West. There's never been a point in history in which humans have been more protected than we are today. This is obviously a huge positive achievement for humankind. But it comes with a cost: many of us are over-reliant on never experiencing any form of discomfort.

▶ This reliance on comfort stops us from pushing ourselves and trying new challenges and, critically, it also stops us from moving our bodies. Most of the chronic diseases we are suffering from these days, including type 2 diabetes, can be directly tied to our reliance on comfort. Lack of movement also makes us more susceptible to cancer, obesity, heart attacks and strokes.

▶ The reliance on comfort also causes us stress. The modern world, with all the efficiency and convenience it offers, gives us an unrealistic expectation that we can always get what we want, when we want it. This is a reliance that can easily and regularly cause problems for us, because we then end up experiencing stress and irritation when even the slightest of things go wrong.

▶ Breaking the reliance on comfort means giving our brains the signal that we have the resilience to cope with ordinary experiences of discomfort. This is why practices like Spartan Races, Tough Mudders, Ultramarathons, Breath Hold Work and wild swimming can have huge psychological benefits. But we don't need to go to extreme lengths to break this reliance; fasting, cold showers, parkruns, wild camping, a morning routine or simply trying something new that will stretch us somehow can also be very effective.

▶ Creating your own personal list of "discomfort rules" – like always taking the stairs – will get you away from constant decision-making and help make choosing discomfort your default way of being.

5. TAKE LESS OFFENSE

Reliance on being right

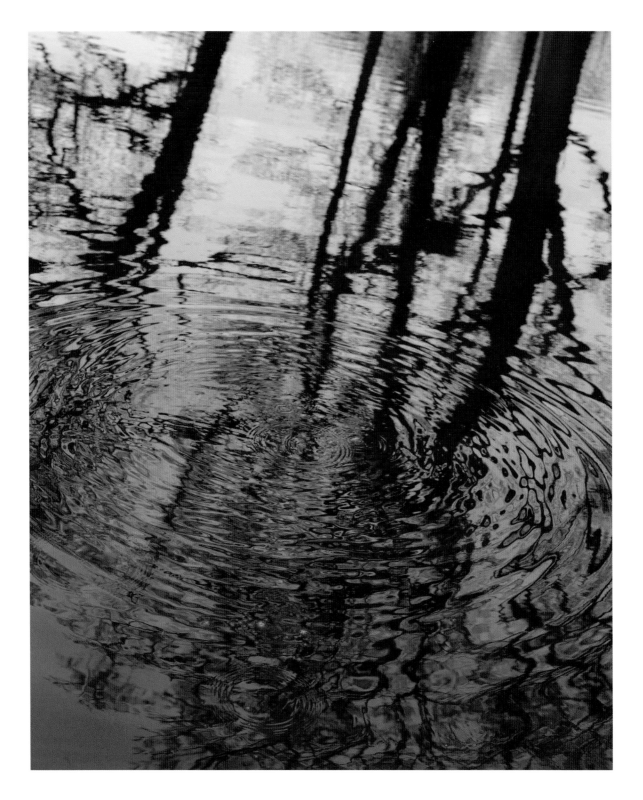

The days after the death of George Floyd, in May 2020, were tense on both sides of the Atlantic. Coming in the midst of a psychologically taxing lockdown, the event had a heightened impact on millions of people and began a fresh conversation on the state of race relations in the West. I am from a family of Asian immigrants that has, over the years, on occasion, had to deal with certain levels of discrimination in the UK. In the immediate aftermath of Floyd's death, I decided not to post a rushed and ill-thought-out response, instead meditating on the issue for a couple of days before adding my voice to the conversation in a careful and considered way. In a post on Instagram, I described some of the racism my wife had experienced when she was a young girl. One night, her family had a brick thrown through their living room window by a local extremist group. In my post, I described from my perspective the impact that racism can have.

Almost immediately, I received an aggressive and vitriolic response from certain people on social media. I was told in no uncertain terms that this was a "Black" issue, and it was not my turn to talk about "Asian" experiences. I'll admit that my immediate response was panic. Had I unwittingly undermined the Black community in their time of pain? Should I make an apology video and promise to "do better"? But the panic quickly faded. I hadn't signed up to any code of conduct that dictated how I should or should not respond to this tragedy. The furor around it led to a few days of deep reflection for me, which I chose to share with my followers, exactly as I was entitled to do. But a significant number of people chose to take offense at what I'd written.

Note: In this chapter I am using the word "triggered" to indicate the more colloquial use of the term. Traditionally, the word was reserved for mental health circles and referred to trauma, generally describing certain words, events, sounds or experiences that would "trigger" a person's body and mind to react as if they were still in harm's way, even if they were not. Colloquially, the term "triggered" is now also used to refer to a strong internal emotional reaction in response to someone else's words or actions. This is how I am using the word in this chapter.

A TWENTY-FIRST-CENTURY SUPERPOWER

I realize, naturally, that I am far from alone in this experience. There are more than 4 billion people on social media – around half the population of the world – so it's no exaggeration to say that at least hundreds of millions of us will have received aggressive, intolerant responses from strangers about things we've posted. Not only is this upsetting to those who are recipients of this negativity, it is also going to have a detrimental effect on those who have chosen to take offense in the first place. Sadly, a tendency to police the beliefs and behaviors of others is so common it appears to be part of our nature. But just because this instinct is part of our nature, it doesn't mean we have to be prisoner to it. We can choose to mindfully become more accepting, and take offense less often, if we wish.

If you think that taking less offense is only really important for people who are always online, I'd invite you to think again. How many bitter arguments between friends, colleagues and loved ones have taken place because someone has taken offense to something another person has said or done? Now consider these dynamics on a larger scale. How much mistrust and hatred has been generated between people of different races, religions, cultures and social classes, because they see the world differently? I hope you can appreciate that this is not just an issue for people who spend too long on their phones – although it does matter a good deal for them. If everybody on the planet devoted a small amount of time each day to the exercises in this chapter, the sum of human mistrust, violence and hatred would plummet. If I could choose one improvement that I could cast, like a magic spell, on the population of the world it wouldn't be to do with exercise or diet or sleep, it would be this: taking less offense.

THE EGOTISTICAL RELIANCE

When you dig down into it, there's a crazy level of arrogance that's needed for us to seriously take offense. It means we believe the person whose words or actions we have taken offense to has no right to a different perspective. In effect, what we're saying is that in this incredibly diverse world we live in, filled with people who have an almost endless array of different cultures, histories, traditions, preferences and beliefs, there should really be just one way of seeing the world – our way. When you see it laid out like this, it sounds insane. And yet many of us are guilty of thinking like this, sometimes multiple times a day. Our reliance on wanting everyone in the world to agree with everything we think is a massive yet normalized problem.

Taking less offense is about much more than just allowing us to get on better with each other. I genuinely believe that training ourselves to be less offended is one of the most important things we can do for our physical, mental and emotional health. To understand why, it's important to know how the way we perceive things affects the nervous system. Imagine you receive an email from your boss that you decide to interpret as rude and confronting. The moment you do that, your nervous system will respond: signals will shoot out around your brain and body that communicate that you're suddenly under threat. This is a system that evolved tens of thousands of years ago, when we were evolving in a hunter-gatherer context and threats were genuinely things that had the potential to kill us, whether a saber-toothed tiger or an invading tribesman.

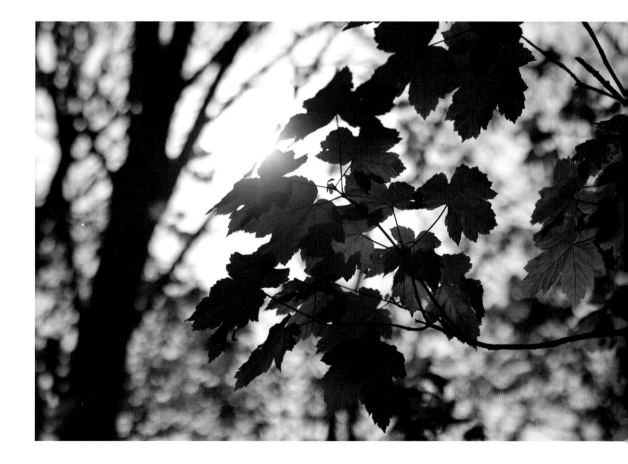

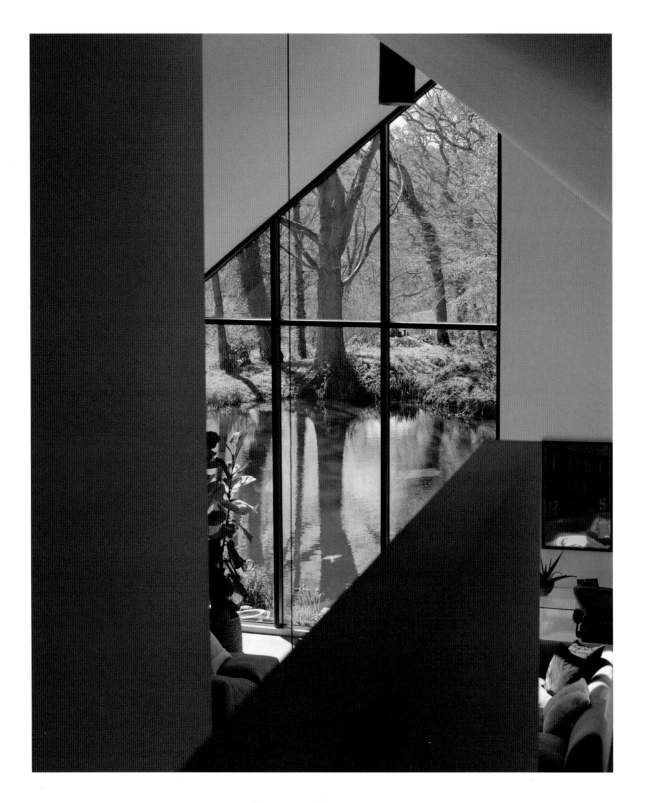

To your subconscious, it doesn't matter exactly what has happened – a threat is a threat. When you read that email, as far as your nervous system is concerned, there is a spear coming at your head. It primes you to focus all your energy and focus towards the incoming danger and to deal with it with a level of ferocity that, in most cases, just isn't appropriate for a twenty-first-century environment. When our nervous system is on high alert like this, it can be incredibly difficult for us to respond rationally. It literally changes the way we experience reality. We become hypervigilant, looking out for threats all around us. When this happens, we struggle to see the big picture – in that moment, the big picture is irrelevant. We become self-interested, less tolerant and less empathetic. The brain wants us to overreact in this way because, tens of thousands of years ago, overreaction would have given us the best chance of survival. But overreacting to our bosses, friends, loved ones or strangers on the internet will most likely do nothing but trigger an aggressive reaction from them in response. In the end, everyone becomes irrational and aggressive because the nervous systems of all involved are firing on all cylinders.

Living too much in this heightened mode is a major upstream problem for our health. It switches our body into its stress state, in which inflammation is increased. When we spend too long in this state, we become more vulnerable to a host of potentially life-threatening diseases, including cancer, heart disease, type 2 diabetes and bowel disorders like ulcerative colitis and Crohn's disease. It's also terrible for our general wellbeing. When we send signals to ourselves that we're constantly under threat from other people, we feel out of control, and seek out compensatory behaviors. For example, we may find ourselves trying to soothe our emotional stress by having a bit more sugar or an extra glass of wine after work. To put it simply, if we're vulnerable to taking offense, we're unable to thrive.

Once we develop the skill of not taking offense – and it is not as hard as we might initially think – we set off a very powerful ripple effect. Because we now don't interpret that email or comment or social media post as threatening in the first place, we don't end up activating our stress state, which means we are generating less internal tension. This, in turn, means that we are much less likely to feel the need to overconsume substances, like sugar, alcohol and caffeine. It also means that, over time, our perception of the world becomes more forgiving, accepting and calm.

Of course, learning not to take offense is more difficult for some people. Many of us have experienced traumatic events in life, which have programmed our nervous systems to react in specific ways, in response to certain events or "triggers." For these people, it can be more challenging to consciously change their responses. But it's not impossible. Without question, therapy with a trained healthcare professional can be helpful but, unfortunately, not everyone has access because of availability and cost. Even without it, though, there is much that we can do ourselves, and the tools in this chapter will still help.

ADOPT A LEARNER MINDSET

When was the last time you took offense to something somebody else said or did? When we understand what's really going on when we take offense, it's clear that it's not really possible for anyone else to offend us. It is our nervous system that is reacting, generating the response, not anybody else's. The fuse that is being lit resides within us. When we place the blame elsewhere, we give power to other people – even complete strangers on the internet. If we want to thrive, we must give up our reliance on blaming the external world for our own internal responses.

One of the single most powerful things we can do to rewire our responses is to adopt the mindset of a learner. Just imagine someone is bothering you. You feel emotionally triggered by some of the things they've said. It is worth stopping for a moment and asking yourself, why am I choosing to take offense? What might this situation look like if I didn't?

A lot of the time, we feel aggressive and defensive towards a person because we are trying to protect a fragile identity we have built up for ourselves. It becomes extremely important to defend this identity by always being right. In fact, our subconscious mind wants us to be right so much that we go about each day looking for any evidence we can find that will support our existing beliefs. When we come across someone with a different viewpoint, it threatens our identity and when we cling on to our identities too tightly, we become fragile. We become prone to being offended all the time, which is bad for us emotionally, physically and socially. Why socially? Because the reality is that most people find it pretty exhausting being around people who are always angry and complaining.

Adopting the mindset of a learner switches us out of this defensive mindset. It gives us freedom from the reliance on always being right. If our basic approach is

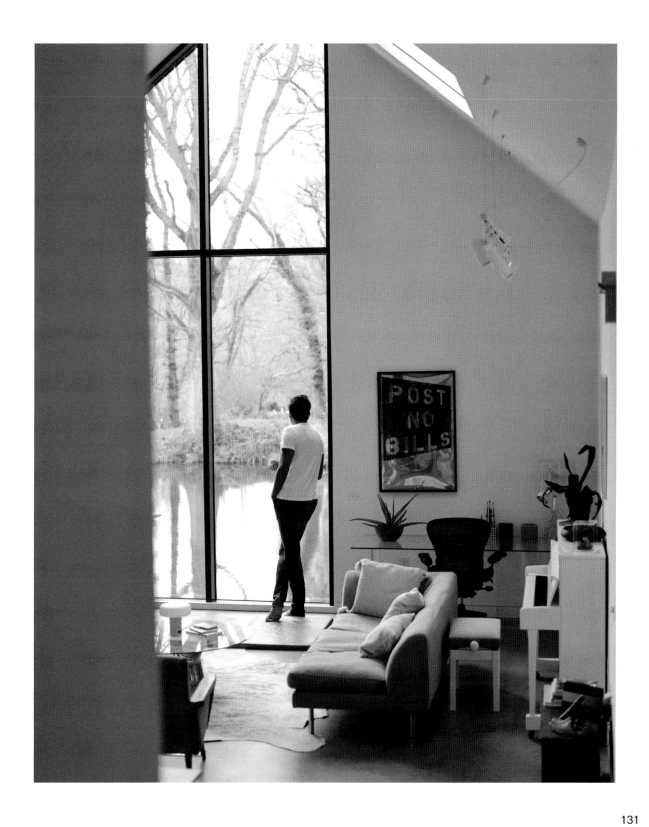

to figure out what is true, rather than to prove that all our opinions and ideas about the world are always correct, our lives will be transformed. We will see rapid improvements in our personal relationships, work relationships, the quality of the time we spend on social media, and our health. I genuinely believe this is one of the most effective changes that I have made in my own life over the past few years, and is one of the main reasons I feel so happy, calm and content these days. Since I let go of the reliance on being right, the world has become a more peaceful and beautiful place. Every day feels like a school day, in the best possible way. If I find myself getting annoyed at someone and disagreeing with what they are saying, instead of trying to push them into changing their opinion, I try to imagine what has led to them having their alternative view. It is perfectly possible to choose not to take offense and, instead, choose empathy and compassion.

It's common for people to confuse not taking offense with putting up with problematic behavior. This is a complete misunderstanding. When you train yourself to not take offense, you keep your nervous system in a calm state and keep your emotional cool, which in turn means you are better able to change things that you do not like. If the email you received from your boss is creating friction, not taking emotional offense to it will mean you are much better able to have a rational conversation with them about it. The same goes for everything in life. Not getting triggered enables you to make meaningful change more effectively.

THE IDENTITY TRAP

The main reason that so many of us walk around with a reliance on being right is because we have built up fragile identities that crack under the slightest bit of pressure. Unless we become mindful of them, they can easily become a problem. But what exactly is an identity? You could think about it as a kind of "off the peg" person that we try to dress up in. We all have an idea what a "doctor," an "environmentalist," a "soccer player" or a "banker" is. When we join these tribes, we dress up in their identities. But identities can be a trap. They can keep us limited. They can also brainwash us into believing that one particular worldview is always correct, while all others are invalid and in need of correction. Many of us don't know what we actually think any more. We confuse the thoughts of our identity-tribes with our own views. When this happens, we call it "groupthink." This is a trap that

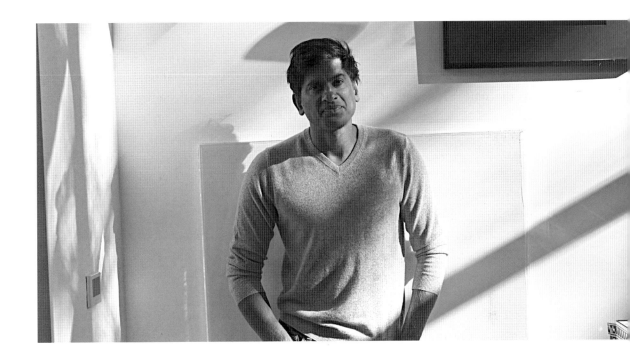

many of us are constantly falling into and is especially common with people who spend a lot of time on social media.

For the past few years, I have been taking progressively longer social media vacations each summer. It started off as seven days; last year it ended up being six weeks. One of the things I love most about these breaks is that they give me the space to reconnect with my own beliefs, without just taking on those of the world around me.

Many of us are blissfully unaware of how much our views and perspectives are shaped by external forces. This is especially true in the online world, where we tend to follow people and read articles that we like and whose opinions we already agree with. The social media platforms also reinforce this pattern by repeatedly showing us content they think we are going to like, which typically means content that aligns with our own existing views. It's easy to fall into the trap of thinking that everyone else around us sees life in exactly the same way as we do. Then, when we do get exposed to a different worldview, it threatens our identity. But what has actually happened? Nothing. Someone just happened to have a different viewpoint. That is all.

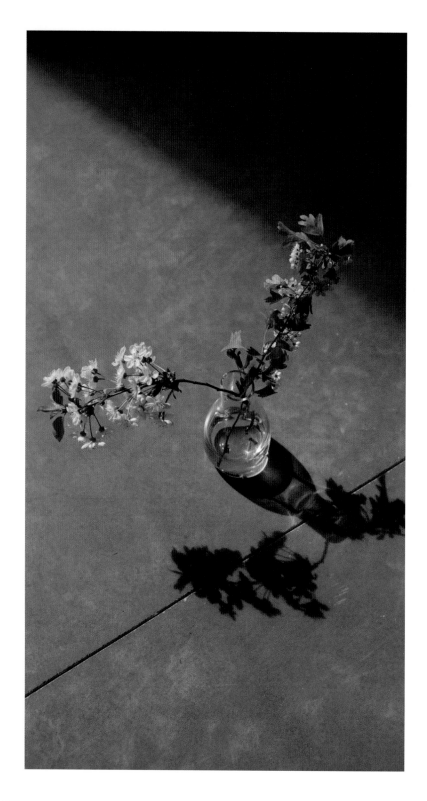

Over the last few years, I have noticed that a lot of people have a huge part of their identity wrapped up in how they choose to eat. They have found what works for them, which is great. But this doesn't necessarily mean it is going to be right for everyone else. If anyone recommends a different way of eating, their default position is that the other person is "wrong." They struggle to get their heads around the idea that another person in this world of 8 billion people has experienced an improvement in their health by eating in a different way to them. But this is a trap that people typically only fall into if the way they eat has become a part of their identity.

When are you over-reliant on protecting your identity? When do you get triggered if someone else thinks differently to the way that you do? Once you become aware of where these identity traps exist in your own life, you immediately become empowered to change things. You let go of your reliance on being right and immediately the world becomes a kinder, friendlier and calmer place.

FIVE SIMPLE WORDS TO NAVIGATE TRICKY CONVERSATIONS

I have a phrase I use that has proved incredibly helpful for navigating tricky conversations. Not only does it help you take less offense to others, it also results in others taking less offense to you. Rather than saying, "That's not right" or "I disagree," try saying the following five words instead:

▶ "I have a different perspective."

It sounds simple but, believe me, it's astonishingly powerful. It works because it removes the element of personal challenge and implies a horizontal rather than vertical relationship with the person you're talking to. Basically, it allows you to keep chatting as equals, without any party feeling threatened.

It also allows you to continue your dialogue without making the other person "wrong." It says, "Yes, I hear you. That is interesting. I actually see that situation differently." It's a phrase that has curiosity and compassion at its heart and has been transformative in my marriage.

I'd like to challenge you to start using this phrase regularly whenever you come across disagreement or someone who has a different opinion to you. You can use it with your partner, your kids, your friends, your work colleagues, your family and in any online conversations. If you only take one piece of practical advice from this chapter, I'd like it to be this one.

I am certain that once you start using this phrase regularly, you will start to experience life differently. You'll feel calmer, less stressed, and the quality of your relationships will improve, as well.

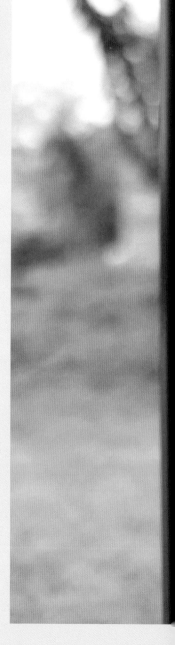

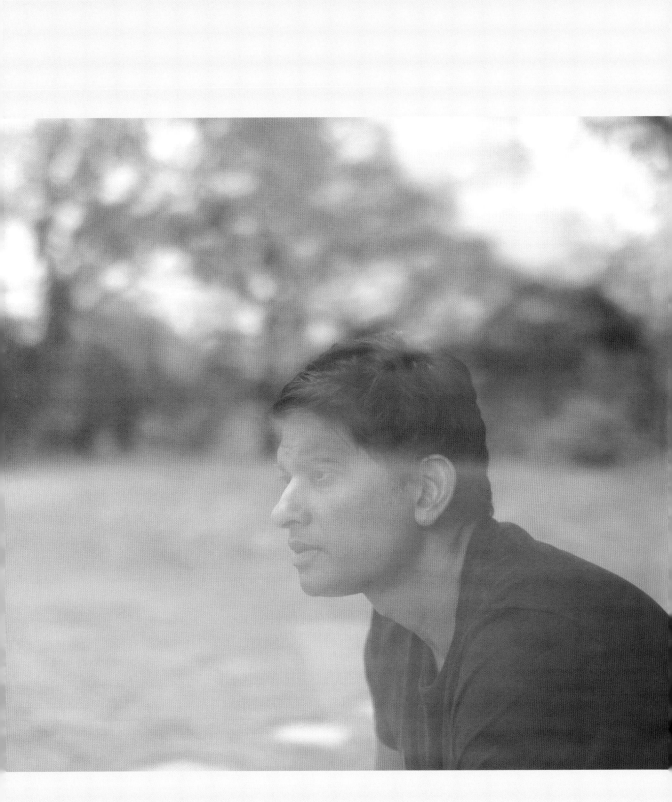

IT'S OK TO NOT KNOW

If we want to let go of our reliance on being right, we need to become friends with these three magic words: "I don't know." So many of us are petrified of uttering these words because we think that people will think less of us. But this is simply not true. When we have the courage to say, "I don't know," we bring people closer to us. They trust us more, respect us more and are drawn to our humility, vulnerability and authenticity.

Unfortunately, the fear of saying "I don't know" is widespread in society. Over the last two decades I have seen first-hand the damage this reliance on being right has done in my own world of medicine. It is not uncommon these days to hear from patients who say they do not feel heard by their doctors. There are, of course, many

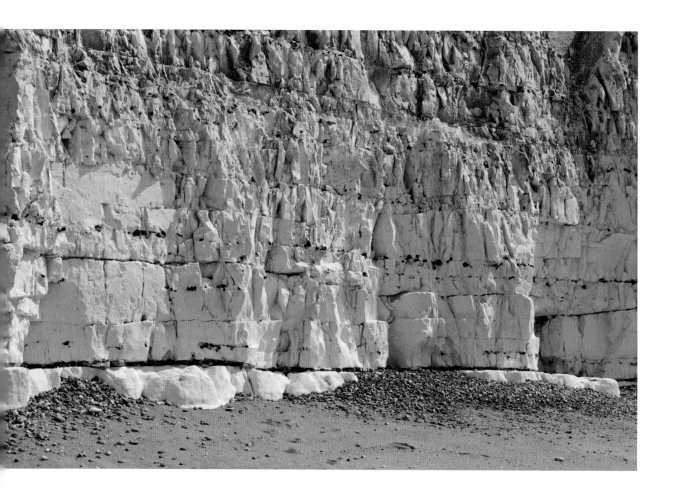

different reasons for this, not least the very short consultation times. However, a crucially important but underappreciated cause lies in our innate desire as humans to be right, or at least to feel right. And doctors are not immune from this.

Research suggests that between 25 and 50 percent of symptoms presenting to doctors are medically unexplained. This means, on many occasions, despite all of our training and expertise, we may not be able to give patients a true answer as to what's going on with them. But doctors are just like everybody else. They have their own insecurities and often try to maintain their identities by giving the impression that they always know what is causing a patient's symptoms. The very best doctors I know have often said to me something along the lines of "the more patients I see, the more I realize how much I don't know." They know what they know, but they are also very aware of what they don't know. And when we are secure enough in ourselves to admit when we don't know something, we give ourselves permission to keep learning. Not only that, we give that permission to those around us. I don't think it's any coincidence that these same doctors are the ones who seem less stressed and calmer than those who are overly reliant on being right. As the psychologist and author Adam Grant writes in *Think Again*: "If knowledge is power, knowing what we don't know is wisdom."

All of us, no matter who we are or where we are on our life journey, will benefit from saying these three magic words more often. When you say these words with compassion and humility, you will find that you have closer and more intimate relationships with others, and with yourself.

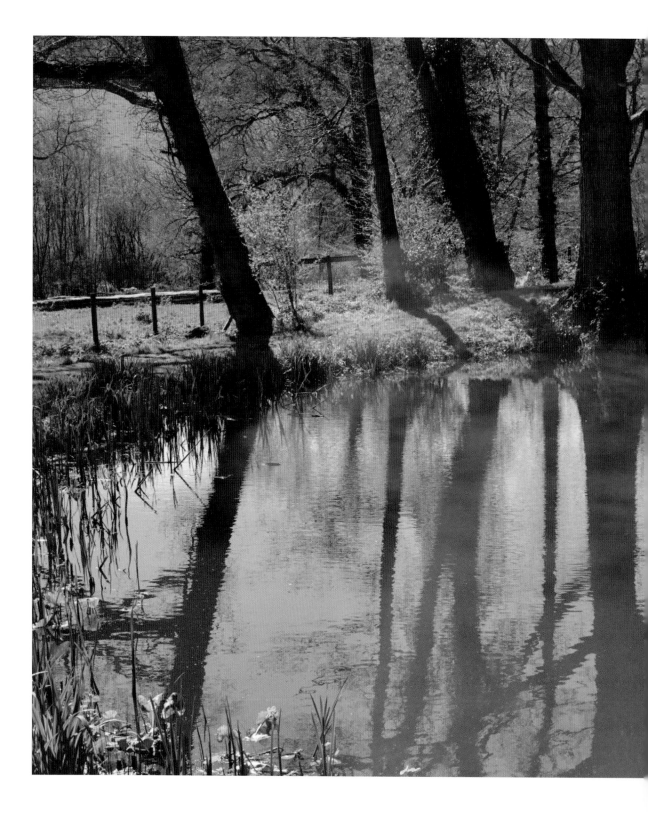

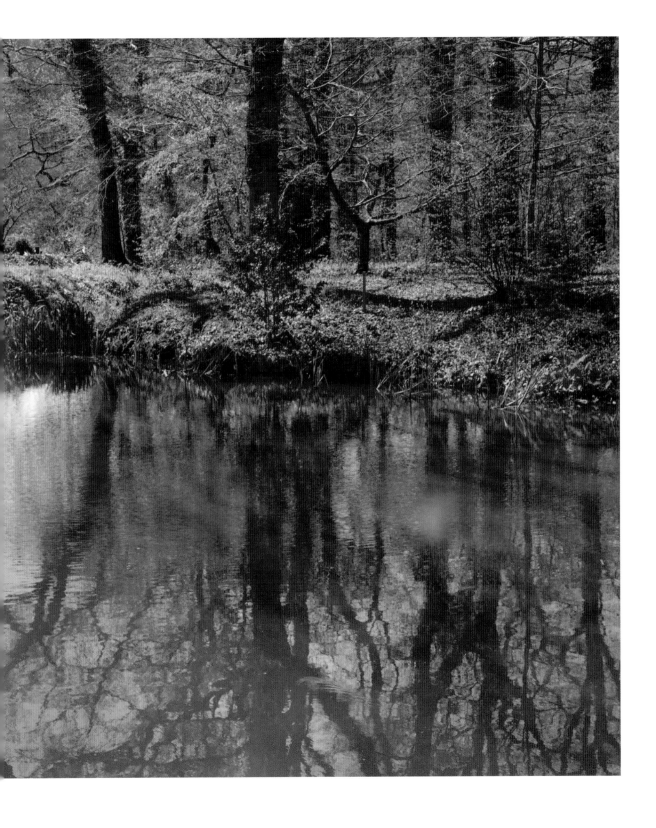

EMBODY CURIOSITY
EVERY DAY

I've written in my previous book *Happy Mind, Happy Life* about the importance of living in alignment with our personal values. It's critical for our health, happiness and our relationships. At this stage in my life, my three most important values are integrity, compassion and curiosity.

Over the last few months, I've come to the realization that curiosity may well be the highest value of all. When we are curious, we naturally act with more compassion and integrity. If our default approach is always to find out more, we're automatically more empathetic towards other people and viewpoints, and this in turn helps us live a life of integrity.

If you find yourself taking offense too often, I'd encourage you to try this delightfully simple practice. In all of your daily interactions, see if you can approach them with a mindset of curiosity.

► Perhaps someone pushes in front of you in a line, and you initially don't like it. Approach this situation not with outrage but curiosity. I wonder what might be going on for that individual. Did they see me? Were they tired? What else might explain what happened?

► Next time your boss sends you an email that you decide to interpret as rude, ask yourself, what might be going on in their life? Why might they be sending an email with this tone? Or, could it be that you have misinterpreted the email because of how you are feeling at the moment?

► If someone has a different opinion to you, instead of judging it as right or wrong, use it as a trigger for inquiry. What life experience has caused them to have this belief? Might we be able to update our own views because of something new we have learned? And might there be a chance that they are actually right, and we are wrong?

You can literally do this anywhere, at any time, in any situation. If you make curiosity your initial goal, you will find yourself becoming calmer and more content immediately.

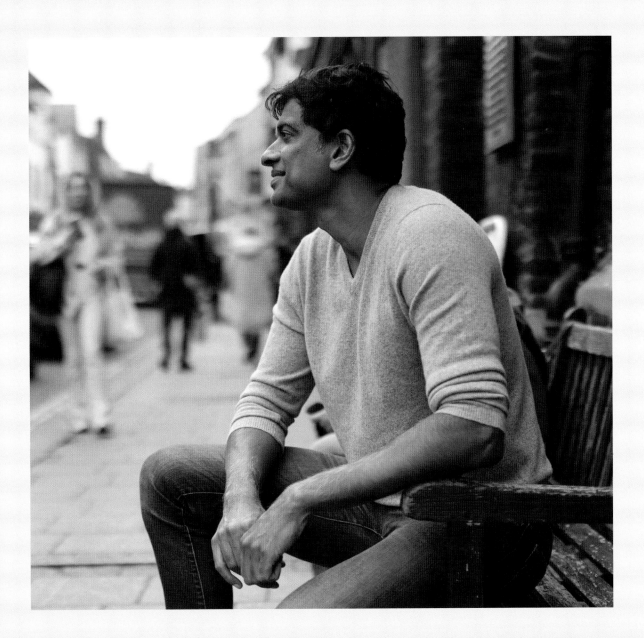

BLACK-AND-WHITE THINKING

One of the main reasons so many people default to taking offense is because they fall into the trap of black-and-white thinking. This can be especially true when we find ourselves on the receiving end of criticism. When I was at university, I remember one occasion when I went back home for the vacations, having maybe enjoyed a bit too much of the good life, and my mum said to me, "What have you been doing? You look fat." Because this was my mum, and I knew it was coming from a place of pure love and concern, I never took offense. Instead, I took her criticism as a genuine signal that I needed to take action, by eating a bit more healthily and drinking a bit less. I had no doubt in my mind that this was exactly my mum's purpose in saying what she did. In fact, in the Indian culture in which I was raised, this type of behavior and directness is the norm.

If I was carrying more weight than I was comfortable with today, how would I feel if a stranger or colleague or someone on social media told me the same thing? A few years ago, I would have no doubt felt annoyed, emotional and offended. I would have told myself a story that the other person has no right to talk about my appearance and that they should know better. But, these days, I wouldn't react like that. I would not fall into the trap of black-and-white thinking by rejecting it immediately and allowing negative thoughts about the other person to creep in. I would try my best to stay emotionally neutral and ask myself if there was any truth to what that person was saying. If there was, I could use their criticism as motivation. If there wasn't, I could simply move on and get on with my day.

Of course, it would be extremely easy for me to get side-tracked into an internal debate about whether that person should be commenting on my appearance. I might find myself phoning a friend to gossip about how out of order they were. I could ruminate over the issue and allow myself to get annoyed and frustrated. But at what cost? What good would any of this actually do? What would it really change? All I would have done is generate emotional stress and inner turmoil that would need to be neutralized in some way or another. Does responding negatively help me or harm me?

It's important that we don't automatically accept or reject the views of other people. When we're being criticized, we could be receiving valuable information. It might be that it has taken our critic a lot of courage and love to speak up. As with my mum,

"The uncomfortable truth is that criticism only bothers us to the extent that we believe it to be true."

their comments might come from a place of deep love and compassion and be a signal that this person cares deeply for us. On the other end of the spectrum, it might be that this person does have malicious intent for us. For whatever reason, they might want to harm us personally or damage our reputation. Sometimes it might be a bit of both; our critic might not wish us well, but that doesn't mean what they're saying is entirely false.

The uncomfortable truth is that criticism only bothers us to the extent that we believe it to be true. If I believe, for example, that I have actually put on a bit of weight, the criticism from others alerting me to this bothers me because I know deep down that what they are saying is correct. Instead of taking responsibility and dealing with the actual issue, it is much easier to put the blame on the person who is dishing out the criticism. In that way, we can avoid dealing with the real issue.

I completely understand that listening to criticism is something that we naturally find emotionally difficult. I used to as well. But it is absolutely possible to change this with consistent, intentional practice and you will find that your ability to thrive will be massively improved when you do. Let go of your reliance on never hearing negative comments about yourself. And, instead, use them as an opportunity to learn – whether that learning is something you can use to improve yourself or whether it is simply that the criticism says more about the other person (and their beliefs and state of mind) than about you.

Note: In this section above, I am not referring to situations involving physical and/or emotional abuse.

WIDEN THE GAP

The next time you find yourself wanting to take offense at something, see if you can take a pause. You might be able to work through the situation in your mind right there in the moment; if not, turn it into a journaling exercise towards the end of the day.

Either way, go through the following step-by-step process to help you gain clarity on the situation and your emotions surrounding it:

▶ What is it that is causing you to want to take offense?

▶ What is it specifically that is bothering you?

▶ Is there another way to look at this situation?

▶ Is it the intention of that person to offend you?

▶ What story about the situation could you write in your mind that would add compassion and understanding?

▶ Can you imagine a scenario whereby you would understand why that person has that point of view? For example, their childhood, upbringing, parents, early life experience, friends etc. Does this change how you feel about them?

▶ Is there any possibility that you might have misinterpreted things and got the wrong end of the stick?

▶ What would happen if you did not *choose* to take offense here?

With regular practice, you will find that you feel offended less often and are able to take a different, more empowering perspective in many situations.

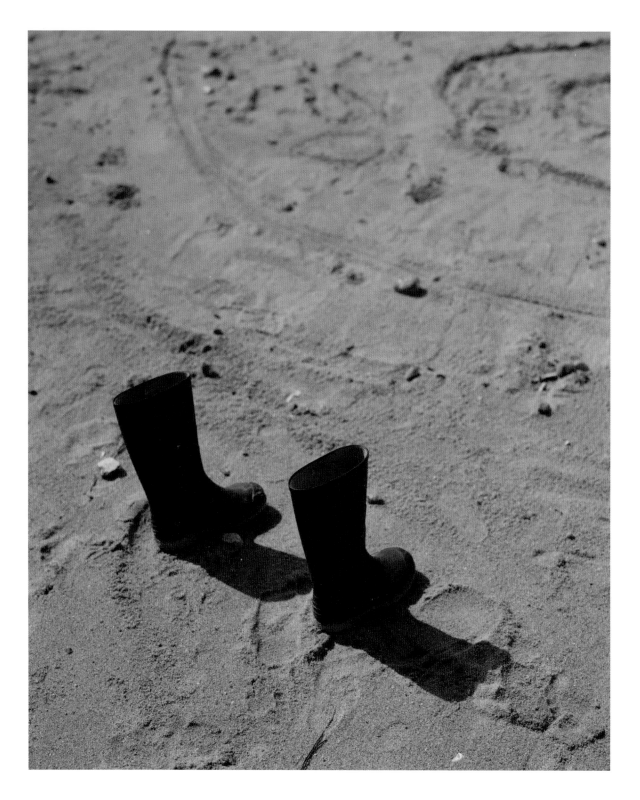

CONCLUSION

▶ Especially since the rise of social media, many of us have developed an unhealthy reliance on always being right. We have also experienced what it's like to be insulted and attacked by people who have a different perspective to us. But the reliance on being right doesn't just affect people who spend the majority of their waking hours online. Most of us have fallen out with loved ones over simple disagreements in perspective.

▶ The demand that everyone share our beliefs is unrealistic. Breaking this reliance is not only good for our mental and physical health, it will make us kinder, more accepting and more lovable.

▶ To break this reliance, we can practice our skills of insight. What are the beliefs we have that are so precious that we become irrationally angry and defensive when someone disagrees with them? Why do we feel this way? What, in our past, created this emotional trigger?

▶ We can also adopt a learner mindset. We should embrace curiosity and the practice of saying "I don't know." Our basic approach should be to work out what is true, rather than to prove that all our beliefs are always correct.

▶ The reliance on being right creates stress and increases our risk of mental and physical illness. It also makes us socially isolated. Cutting the reliance will make us calmer, happier and more connected and in control.

6. EXPECT ADVERSITY

Reliance on things never going wrong

Have you ever heard of the theory that we should aim to become "1 percent better" every day? I used to buy into this idea, but over the last few years, I've come to believe it's an unhelpful and potentially damaging concept. The simple fact is that progress is nonlinear. Anyone who runs regularly knows this. You can show up every single day to do the training and go literally weeks without any improvement at all. Some days you even go backwards. But then, apparently out of nowhere, you'll shoot forward in progress and achieve a new personal best. If you're reliant on achieving a new personal best every time you run, even if it's just a tiny improvement of 1 percent, you're going to become disappointed in yourself – and perhaps even disillusioned with running itself.

In Chapter 4 I described my love of Breath Hold Work, the practice of intentionally holding my breath. That, too, has a nonlinear path to improvement. In those pages I told you that after my initial four-week course, I managed to increase the time I could hold my breath from one minute to four minutes twenty seconds. Sounds good, doesn't it? But this morning I only managed one minute fifty-five seconds. Why? Because my mind was on this book! I wasn't able to stay calm and centered because my head was buzzing with ideas all night and I didn't sleep well. I just wanted to get my practice over with so I could begin writing. But does that mean it wasn't worth doing. Not at all.

If you're reliant on seeing evidence of progress every day in order to motivate you to do more, you are going to struggle. Even if you are on the right weight loss plan, the number on your scales will not go down every single day. Even if your marriage is thriving, there will be days you have to navigate conflict. Even if you are progressing with a piano piece you are learning, it will not sound amazing every time you play it.

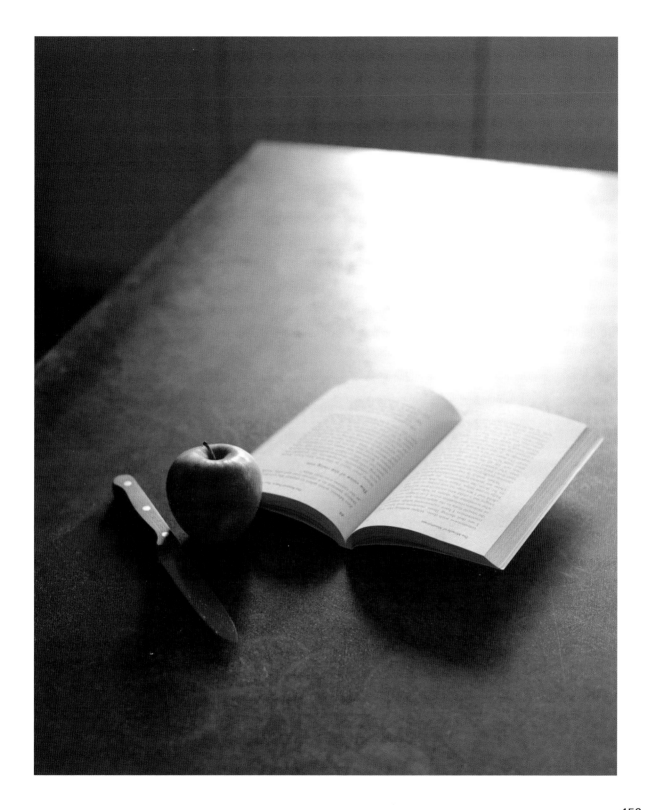

None of this means you are failing. The fact is, you're not the same person every day. Some days you're on your game, on other days you're not. And even when things are getting better, they're also going to get worse. Ups are always interspersed with downs. Nonlinear progress is practically a law of the universe. It's just how things work.

THE ESCALATOR MYTH

We know, intellectually, that nothing gets better indefinitely, that steps forward are always interlaced with steps backwards. But that's not how we tend to behave. Somewhere inside us, we have a subconscious belief that life ought to be like gliding up an escalator, progressing ever upwardin steady, predictable increments. This is what I call the "Life is an Escalator" myth and it's one of the reasons why the "1 percent better" concept has become so popular – it just feels instinctively true. Many of us are reliant on the idea that things will never go wrong, which means we

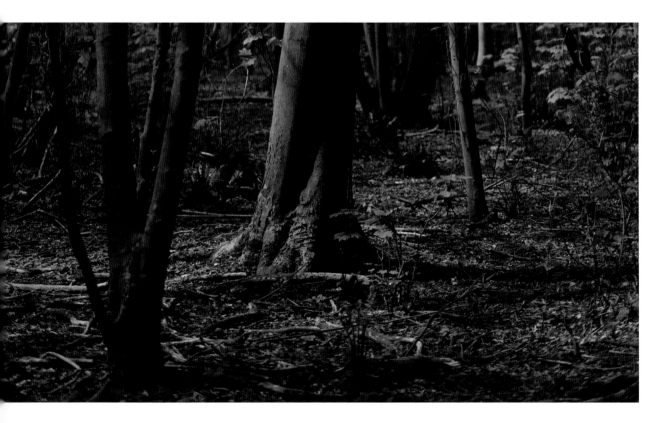

feel frustrated and hard done by when they inevitably do. We're perfectly able and even willing to predict failure and disaster for others, but when bad things happen to us our initial response often takes the form of shock and outrage. "How can this be happening to me?"

The "Life is an Escalator" myth is one of the reasons why people don't check their breasts and testicles for lumps as often as they should. It's why millions of middle-aged people feel betrayed and despairing at the loss of their formerly youthful faces and bodies. It's why drivers break the speed limit on the motorways on days of heavy wind and rain. It's why people happily smoke, vape, binge-drink, eat takeout four times a week and take recreational drugs. It's why, every single year, highly motivated and tough men and women die on the slopes of Mount Everest. They were expecting themselves to hit that incredible peak; it was only other climbers who ever got caught in bad weather or avalanches or accidentally lost their footing and slipped.

Of course, I'd never deny the incredible benefits of being optimistic. How else are we going to have the self-belief necessary to achieve our dreams? But the pure, naive optimism that the escalator myth encourages, can do us a huge amount of damage. If we can only be happy when life plays out in the way we want it to, we'll probably never achieve our dreams. It's far more likely that we'll become disappointed, burnt out and resentful, and then quit going after those dreams altogether.

FACTOR IN YOUR SHRINKAGE

Retail companies around the world have a business concept that I think can be valuable to apply to life in general. That concept is known as "shrinkage." When stores look into the future and work out how much profit they're likely to make, they know they're going to lose a certain amount to factors such as theft, loss and breakage. This loss is their "shrinkage" from the financial position they would've been in if the world was perfect, and nothing bad ever happened to their stock. Shrinkage sets UK retailers back to the tune of around $11 billion a year. This is clearly a huge amount of money but the successful retailers – the ones that end up thriving in the marketplace – are those who accept the inevitable friction of reality and plan for it.

We all have shrinkage waiting for us in our futures. When we look ahead, we can't predict what adverse experiences are coming our way – the only guarantee is that they're coming for us in some form or other. But when we remain reliant on the myth that nothing in our lives will ever go wrong we set ourselves up for misery and sickness.

A close friend of mine was a GP who had a complaint made against them about the misdiagnosis of cancer. The latest statistics show that doctors in the UK will be sued, on average, four times over the course of a forty-year career. This is the standard level of shrinkage any doctor should expect. It doesn't matter how good you are: if you see patients, you are going to get complaints. But even though it was clear from the start that there was no case to answer against my friend, the complaint completely floored him. For the two years that he was investigated he felt constantly stressed, barely slept and drank heavily on weekends. His emotional and physical health went through a slow but steady decline. I understand, of course, that an investigation like this will always be difficult to endure. But the thriving mindset is one that expects adversity and says, "I've been a doctor for two decades and have seen tens of thousands of patients, sometimes in stressful time-pressured consultations. It was inevitable that I would one day be subject to a serious complaint."

My friend's example might appear to be quite an extreme one, but we can apply the same principle to an everyday activity like driving. We could choose to expect that we will never have a crash, or we could look at the odds and accept that if we drive for long enough, there is a strong chance that we will be involved in one at some point. I consider myself a very good driver, and have passed my Institute of Advanced Motorists examination. Despite this, a few months ago, I ended up crashing my car. How did this happen? I was fast asleep when my mum's emergency buzzer went off. I quickly drove over and discovered that she had fallen. I helped her back up, got her settled into bed and once I was happy she was alright left in a hurry to get back to my own bed. I reversed out of her drive in the dark and drove straight into a car that was parked on the opposite side of the road.

If this had happened ten years ago, I would have beaten myself up for days, calling myself an idiot and berating myself for not being more careful. I would also have taken comfort in the victim mindset: "On top of all of this stress with Mum, now I need to sort out the car as well. Why is this happening to me?" Instead, right after

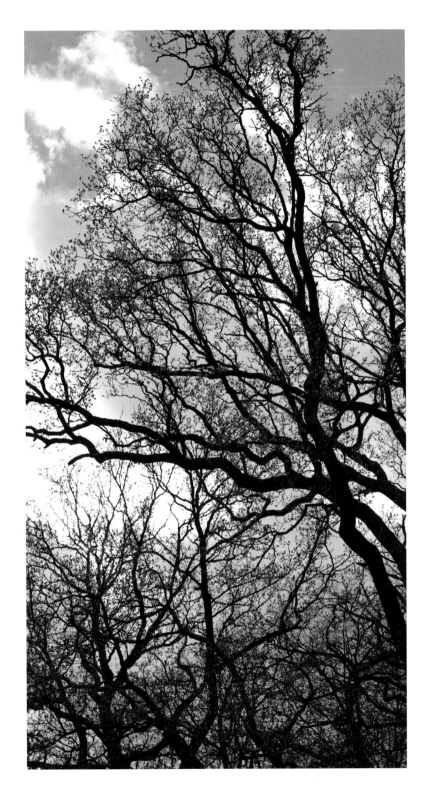

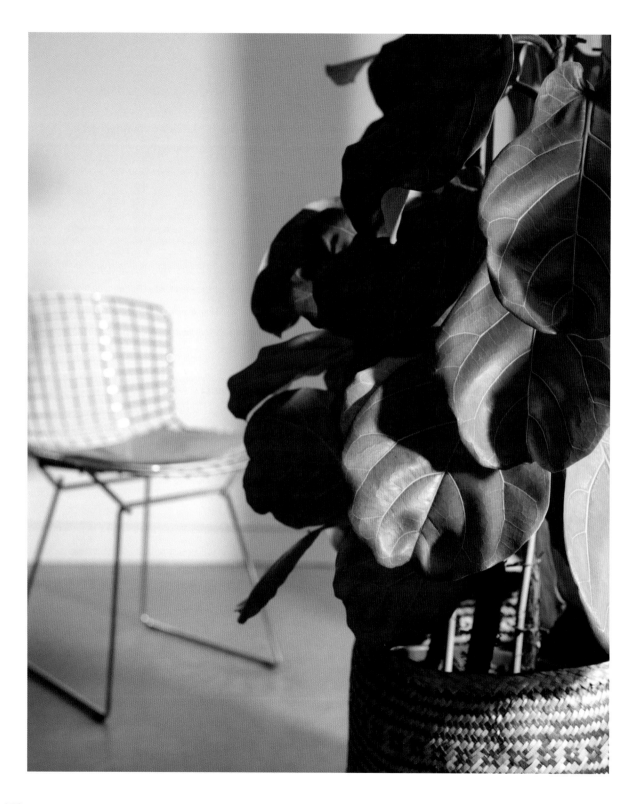

I crashed my car, I neither beat myself up nor fell into the trap of making myself a victim. Because of slow, steady intentional practice over the past few years in Minimal Reliance, my default has started to change. Rather than cursing and feeling sorry for myself, I thought, "Oh well, if you are going to keep coming round to help Mum at night, when you're exhausted and half-asleep, of course something like this was going to happen at some point. In fact, it's amazing it never happened sooner. And, let's be honest, it could have been worse. I'm completely fine. No one got hurt. It's just a car. I have insurance." In other words, I immediately and instinctively accepted the accident as shrinkage.

Life is going to present you with regular opportunities to practice handling adversity. If you commute to work, on some days there will be horrendous traffic or delays, even when you leave in good time. When you nip to the supermarket, there will be times when the person in front of you takes ages and has a long chat with the cashier. One day, your package delivery will arrive when you are not at home and the driver will leave it out to get wet in the rain. How you respond to these events will determine the impact they have on you, and how in control you feel. If you always get frustrated when things do not go your way, you are allowing yourself to be constantly disappointed by the natural order of life. This is irrational. Expecting adversity is about having a realistic model of reality. It's about giving yourself evidence that you can thrive, even when things are going wrong.

THE GIFT OF SHRINKAGE

Where I grew up, in northwest England, most kids at school were either hardcore Manchester United or hardcore Manchester City fans. For years, Manchester City struggled, very much existing in the shadow of their more famous and successful neighbors. But in 2007, a rich new owner bought the club, poured money in and, within years, it became incredibly successful. I remember chatting with friends of mine back then who were diehard City fans. After the initial euphoria, many of them said to me, "We're winning everything all the time, but it's not the same. I preferred it when we only won occasionally. Then every game felt unpredictable and exciting."

For a period of years, Manchester City's success became an escalator. But, as some of the fans found out, it wasn't actually that much fun. It's the same with life. We need the downward parts – the shrinkage – to make the upward parts – the growth – meaningful and enjoyable. The downward parts also teach us and make us stronger. Rather than being an escalator, life is like an accumulator. With every peak climbed and valley crossed, we accumulate strength and wisdom.

THE COMPLAINT SIGNAL

There's a surprisingly easy way of telling if the escalator myth is an invisible reliance that's harming you. Ask yourself honestly, how much do you complain every day? We all complain a little, of course, but the frequency of our complaining can be a clue that this myth has become a problem for us. Whenever we complain about something, we're effectively saying, "I think life should be going a certain way and it's not – and it's X or Y that's standing in my way." It might feel good in the moment, but it doesn't actually serve anyone. Complaining is short-term pleasure for long-term pain, a bit like eating chocolate when you're stressed. It can feel like you're doing something proactive and useful, because your mood has seen a slight improvement, but, if you do this regularly, you're actually setting yourself up for major problems.

For a start, our complaining is not usually enjoyed by the people we share our lives with. They may make sympathetic noises and agree with what we're saying, but if we do it more than a minimal amount, it's not much fun for anyone. It's also a little selfish, like we're peeling off a bit of our negative frame of mind and sticking it on to anyone else who hears us, lightening our load by adding to theirs. But complaining can also harm us by retraining our mind. Think of it like this: whatever we practice in life, we get good at. Just like practicing kick-ups for enough time will make us a better soccer player, complaining all the time will reinforce the idea that life is not going our way and that we're unable to thrive because the world is full of obstacles. With everything we say and do, we create our reality. Complaining is a slow drip of poison to our perception, eating away at our happiness and trust.

One of my favorite people in the world is my father-in-law, Dinesh. After his grandparents sailed to Africa on a tiny boat on a dangerous three-week voyage from India, they settled in Kenya and became successful, middle-class people. Their family set up a candy factory, and Dinesh founded a company that sold designer clothes for kids. But then, in August 1982, the coup took place. There were soldiers going door to door raping and killing people. Vidh herself can viscerally remember, at the age of three, being locked in a cupboard with her brother and told to keep silent because armed men had come to their door. The family lost everything overnight. They moved to the UK where her dad started again from scratch, starting a new business; that failed, so he started a post office and newsagent working seven days a week, from five every morning, for thirty years. Hand on heart, in seventeen years of knowing him I can honestly say I've never once heard him complain about anything. When I ask him about the loss of his businesses, he just smiles and says, "money comes and money goes, it doesn't make you happy."

Vidh's father is every bit as inspirational to me as some of the world-famous people I've spoken to on my podcast. In spite of all the adversity he's experienced, it hasn't broken him or made him bitter or disillusioned. Instead, it's made him free. It's taught him that he has no need to rely on wealth or status to thrive. He's thriving anyway. He truly is a living, breathing example of Minimal Reliance.

Cutting down our complaining is not an example of what's sometimes referred to as "toxic positivity." It doesn't mean pretending that life is perfect. It's about training ourselves to be less reliant on the myth that everything in our lives will always get better. It won't – and that's not actually a bad thing. The trick is to expect adversity, accept it and embrace it. This in turn makes us feel calmer, more resilient and more able to thrive. We should aim to have the mindset described by the Chinese philosopher Lao Tzu, who said, "Never complain, not even to yourself."

REFRAME YOUR COMPLAINTS

The practice that helped me to stop complaining, more than any other, was a simple thought exercise. Every time I heard myself complain about something, without exception, I caught the complaint and reframed it either as a moment of gratitude or a call to action.

▶ If I chose gratitude, I would remind myself how much worse things could be, and how lucky I was in so many other ways.

▶ If I chose action, I would embrace my own power and agency and ability to make the situation better.

Choosing gratitude would stop me *thinking* like a victim. Choosing action would stop me *acting* like a victim.

Both of these "reframes" would reduce my invisible reliances on other people or external events to behave exactly as I wanted them to behave. They would also weaken my reliance on the escalator myth. If you find yourself complaining more than you'd like to, I highly recommend this practice as a powerful way to rewire your thinking.

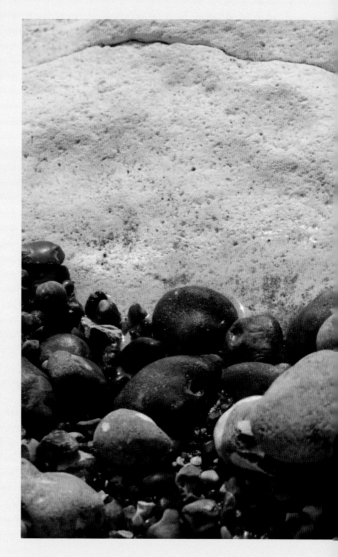

"Choosing gratitude would stop me *thinking* like a victim. Choosing action would stop me *acting* like a victim."

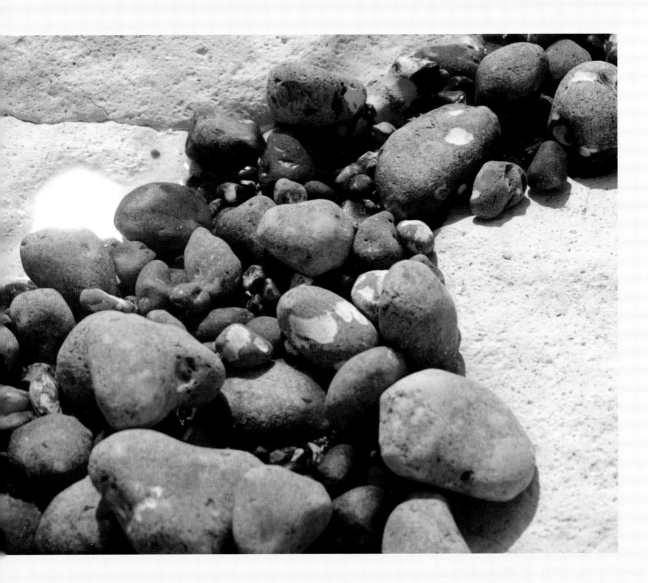

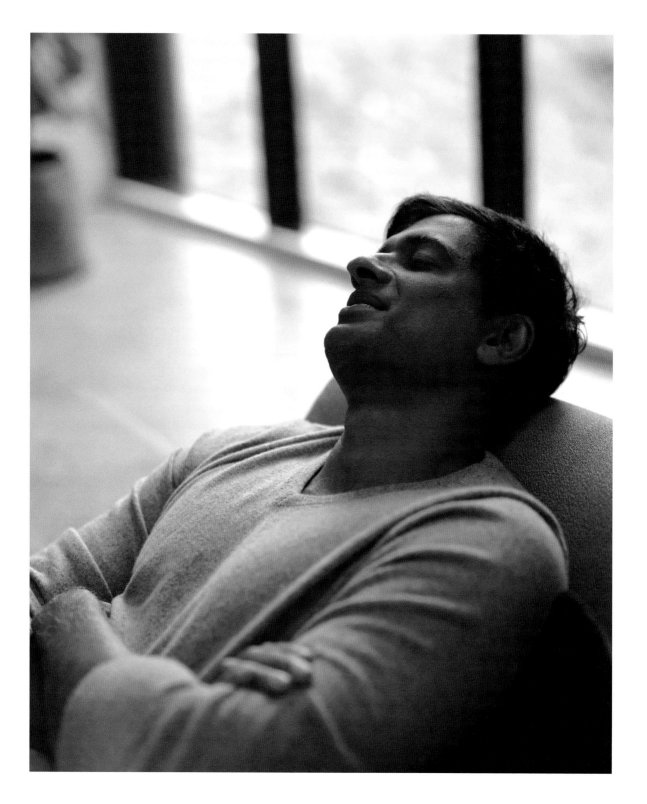

ADVERSITY IN LOVE

The escalator myth is especially damaging to our romantic partnerships. If our close relationships are in bad shape, it is almost impossible to thrive. And yet many of us fall into the trap of expecting our relationships to stay blissful and joyous, with things only ever getting better. This is partly because our culture is flooded with stories of archetypal romance. In books, movies and songs the story is always roughly the same – two lovers meet and after perhaps a rocky start, they realize they are each other's "the one" and live happily ever after. In reality, however, this is rarely ever the case.

Funnily enough, my relationship with Vidh was a little bit like this. Ours was a whirlwind romance. We met on a blind date in 2007 and the attraction was immediate. We went through an incredibly intense and romantic few weeks and I proposed three months after our first date. Five months after that we were married. But that's where the classic, universally recognizable love-story pattern ends. The first year of our marriage was actually incredibly difficult. We had so many arguments and disagreements that we both wondered, more than once, if we had made the right decision. If we hadn't gone and gotten married, we both believe that there's a very high chance we would have gone our separate ways.

But by patiently working through our differences and understanding and accepting each other's perspectives, we came out the other side. I can honestly say, after seventeen years of marriage, that we have never been closer, more committed to each other or happier. The adversity we experienced at the start of our marriage has unquestionably made us stronger.

The fact that relationships can actually be strengthened by stress is well known by relationship experts. In their book *Connect*, David and Carole Robin Bradford write, "Even though conflict can feel stressful and even dangerous, it can actually be very helpful. Conflict can surface issues in a very direct way. It can bring out emotions, indicating what's really going on so you know where others stand." Most people who are in stable, long-term relationships will have experienced this. Successfully managed conflict is what makes you stronger.

Note: For practical tips on how to successfully manage conflict see "How to Have Healthy Conflict" on page 84 and "Five Simple Words to Navigate Tricky Conversations" on page 136.

We naturally want to shy away from adversity. We think it makes our lives less enjoyable. But it is through adversity that we truly find the joy in life. Adversity is also our greatest teacher. It is an unquestionable truth that most of us learn our most powerful lessons by experiencing moments of hardship rather than avoiding them.

"Successfully managed conflict is what makes you stronger."

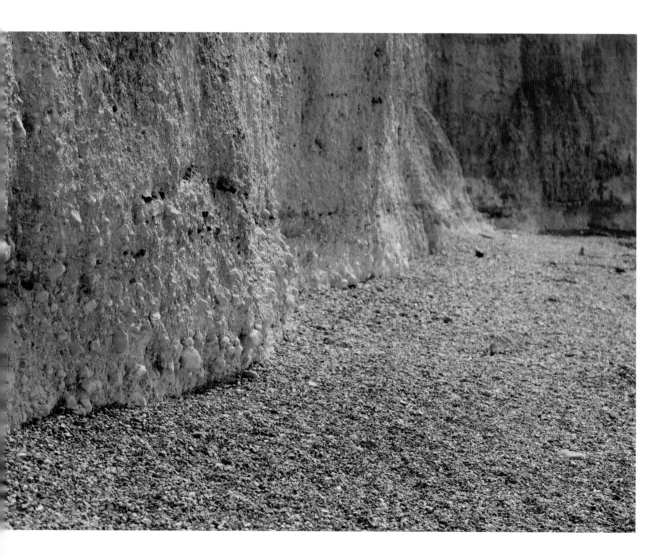

YOU DO NOT COMPLETE ME

Around six years ago, Vidh had an amazing opportunity to go on a week-long course in Germany to help process past traumas, including those that she'd experienced as a girl in Kenya during the coup. It was going to be the longest time she'd ever been away from the family. I was under no illusions about the power of the experience she was about to undergo, and how much it might change her. Before she left, I said to her, "I am so happy you are going on this course. I truly believe this is something you have to do for yourself. If at the end of those seven days, if by processing your past, you change so much that we can no longer be together, I'm completely OK with that. You have to do this for you. I won't resent you one bit. I'll understand."

That was probably the most adult conversation I'd ever had in my life. It left her in tears. But I'm proud that I had the courage and wisdom to say those words. As much as I love Vidh, I'm not reliant on her to make me feel good. I accept that we are two different people who are on our own journeys. I am on my own journey of evolution and so is she. She's free to grow and change – and move on if she has to. And so am I. But, in that lies real beauty. We are coming together consciously. Not because we need to be with each other, but because we want to.

You sometimes hear lovers saying to each other, "You complete me." Sure, it sounds romantic. But I have come to believe that it is deeply unhealthy. I am already complete, and so is Vidh. If we find that we need our partners to complete us, it means we're too reliant on them. This isn't fair on anyone in the relationship. It stops us from thriving. When we're overly reliant on friends and lovers, we stop being ourselves and start being the person we believe they'd prefer. We're more willing to put up with bad behavior from them, and less likely to have the honest conversations that are necessary to keep any long-term relationship healthy.

EXPECTING DEATH

The ultimate form of adversity is death. But Western society hides death from us. Even the language we use around it avoids dealing directly with the subject. We say "they passed" or "I lost someone." But, the uncomfortable truth is, we didn't lose anyone. They died. It isn't like this in India, the country my family originally came from. I have a vague memory from my early childhood of watching the funeral of the Indian prime minister, Indira Gandhi, just days after she had been assassinated. I was only seven years old. I remember us gathering around the television to watch her being placed upon her funeral pyre. We all saw her body go up in flames. It was raw and primal. In India, the fact of death wasn't hidden away politely like it is in Britain. It was right there in your face.

It is only over the past few years that I have begun to reflect on how important images like this can be. For much of my life, I have been afraid of death. When my dad died in 2013 and my two-year-old son asked me where he was, I didn't really know what to say, so I told him, "Dadu has gone up into the sky." These days, I have stopped using these euphemisms around death. I now intentionally say "my dad has died." Not "my dad has passed away" or "I lost my dad." I don't want to tiptoe around it any more. I want to be present with the truth. Facing and embracing his death has helped me hugely; I would say it's one of the main reasons I feel so at peace with it today.

Recently, longevity has become one of the hottest topics in health. On my podcast, I have spoken to experts who believe it is possible to reverse or even completely stop the aging process. Some talk excitedly about humans living for 150 years and longer. I don't want to be someone who stands in the way of innovation and progress, but in our quest for immortality, I'm concerned we're losing sight of something crucially important. Is it not part of the beauty of the human experience that, at some point, it will end?

By not viscerally feeling the reality of death, we develop the unconscious belief that it does not apply to us. We end up taking each day for granted, and labor under the mistaken belief that we have unlimited time to correct what's wrong in our lives. This encourages many of the behaviors, like overwork and not prioritizing our relationships, that can be so toxic to our happiness and health.

This is why I'm determined not to shield my children from the reality of death. Two years ago, my aunt died quite suddenly from cancer. My kids were ten and eight at the time and I didn't want to repeat the mistakes I feel I made when Dad died. In my family's culture, it is customary to have a religious ceremony around the dead body just before the actual funeral, during which the top of the coffin is open so you can see the dead body. Vidh and I discussed whether we should take our children to this ceremony. Would seeing the actual dead body of my aunt be traumatizing? Could they handle it? On reflection, even asking these questions seems a little bizarre. Death is a fundamental part of life. Why are we so desperate to hide it from our children? Is it not better for them to understand and face this reality? We decided to take them to the ceremony because we felt it was important. It was incredibly powerful. Tears were shed, emotions were felt – there was no hiding from it. Death was right there in front of us.

I came to this more enlightened place because my father's death sent me on a journey of grief. As strange as it may sound, it made me realize for the very first time that death really does happen and that the timing of our death is unpredictable and uncontrollable. We could die any day. This should not scare us; it should liberate us. Without death, you cannot experience the beauty of life. Each day is a gift. We can only truly thrive if we appreciate this. Nothing teaches us about the finality of life like death. Nothing teaches us that our possessions are really worthless like death. Nothing teaches us that fame and status ultimately mean nothing like death.

"Without death, you cannot experience the beauty of life."

"Each day is a gift."

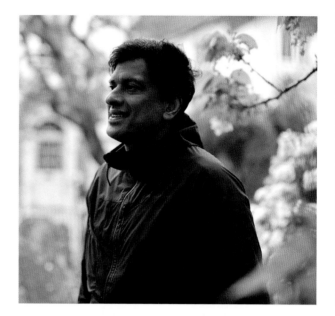

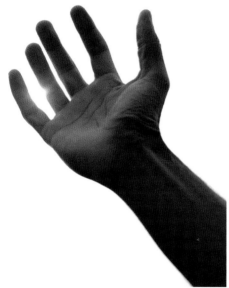

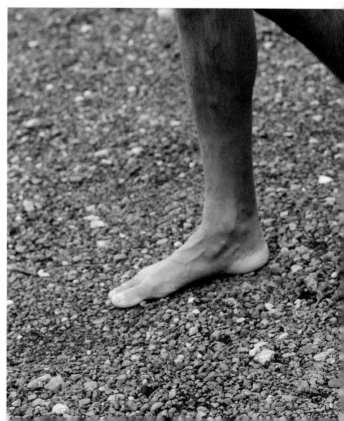

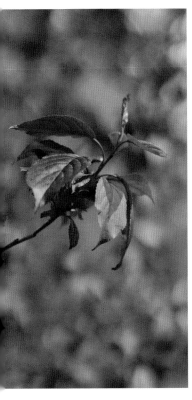

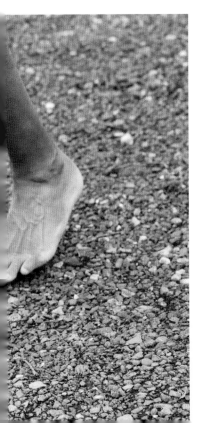

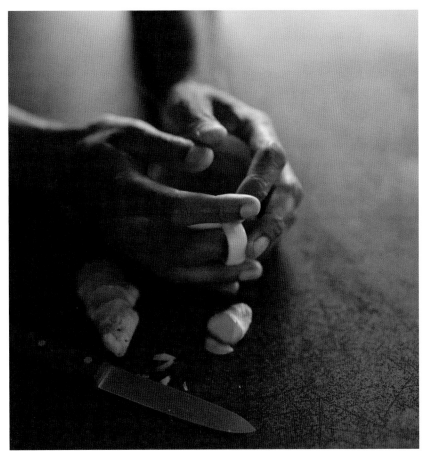

As my journey into grief continued, I began to think about all the things I'd learned and even gained from my father's death. I became my own man through it. I pursued a new career path. And the best thing is, I still have a relationship with him. It's just different now. I can't see my father, but I can still think about him and converse with him in my imagination.

As a result of the journey I've been on, I am no longer afraid of death. One of the insights that helped me most came from the psychology professor Dr. Dacher Keltner, who talked to me on my podcast about the Japanese principle of *wabi-sabi*. It says that the evolution of all forms, whether natural or man-made, always follows a five-stage cycle of creation, birth, growth, decay and death. My discussion with Dr. Keltner was one of the most beautiful conversations I have ever had on my podcast. I was in tears explaining how my mother had changed over the previous months and how I was going through a type of grief for the mum I used to have. Through my reflection on wabi-sabi, I realized that mum was now in the fourth phase, decay. Her body and mind were now decaying and, at some point, in the not too distant future, this decay will turn into death. This is the harsh and brutal truth. It is the natural cycle that has been repeated hundreds of billions of times in the past and will be repeated the same way in the future. Knowing this – and being present with it – has helped me immensely. It has brought me a sense of peace and acceptance. This is the way things are. And, this is the way things will always be. It is who we are.

This deep realization has taught me the importance and beauty of truly appreciating every single moment I have with her. Every single time I leave Mum, I smile with affection and I kiss her on her forehead as I know that one day – soon – it will be the last time.

▶ **To hear more about** *wabi-sabi*, **listen to my conversation with Dr. Dacher Keltner on Episode 340 of my** *Feel Better, Live More* **podcast at drchatterjee.com/340.**

PRACTICE MEDITATING ON DEATH

Psychologists have found a variety of surprising benefits when we regularly reflect on death. Researchers at Eastern Washington University have found that doing so increases gratitude. Another study found that just being physically near a graveyard increases the likelihood that people will help a stranger in need by 40 percent. Reflecting on death has even been shown to make us physically healthier, driving better choices such as reduced smoking and more exercise.

Indeed, many cultures around the world choose to think about death every day in order to enhance their experience of life. For example, some Buddhist monks meditate on death every day as part of their morning routine. If we sit with the knowledge of our own death for a few minutes each morning, it is inconceivable that our approach to the day will not change, even just a little bit.

If you feel that you sometimes take life for granted, I'd encourage you to try the following simple practice. It only takes a few moments but, when done regularly, the benefits can be profound.

▶ As soon as you wake up, spend a moment breathing in bed with your eyes closed. Forget your to-do list, center yourself in your body and reflect on the reality of your death.

▶ Remind yourself that the day you're about to start is not guaranteed. You might fall down dead before your first cup of tea. You may get knocked down by a bus on the way to work. Just acknowledging this to yourself can foster a real sense of gratitude and appreciation for life.

▶ Now, open your eyes, and with your heightened sense of gratitude, you can now proceed with your day.

I personally find this practice really clears the lens and starts to break down the story we tell ourselves that death does not apply to us.

CASE STUDY

A few years back, I had a 52-year-old patient named Brian. He had long-standing issues with his weight and difficulty sleeping. More recently, he had started to develop high blood pressure. It had been clear to me for many years that he was working far too hard. This resulted in him neglecting his marriage, friendships and health. But, no matter what I said, he always seemed reluctant to change.

During one consultation, he told me that he had just seen on Facebook that one of his childhood friends had died suddenly from a heart attack. It hit him really hard. I suggested that he begin the practice of actively thinking about death. For three minutes each morning, he was to remind himself that he was a human being who some day was going to die.

Over the next few months, he slowly realized that he didn't want to work so hard any more. He began to understand that he already had more than enough in his life. The things he'd wished for as a 19-year-old had all happened. Yet, he had always been unable to appreciate what he had and continued pushing for more. Now, with this new insight, he started leaving work on time, so he could spend more time with his family. He also turned down a big promotion. Over the next few months, his blood pressure came back down to normal, his sleep improved and he effortlessly started to lose weight. He also felt much closer to his wife and his vitality for life quickly returned. By regularly thinking about death, Brian had finally started to live.

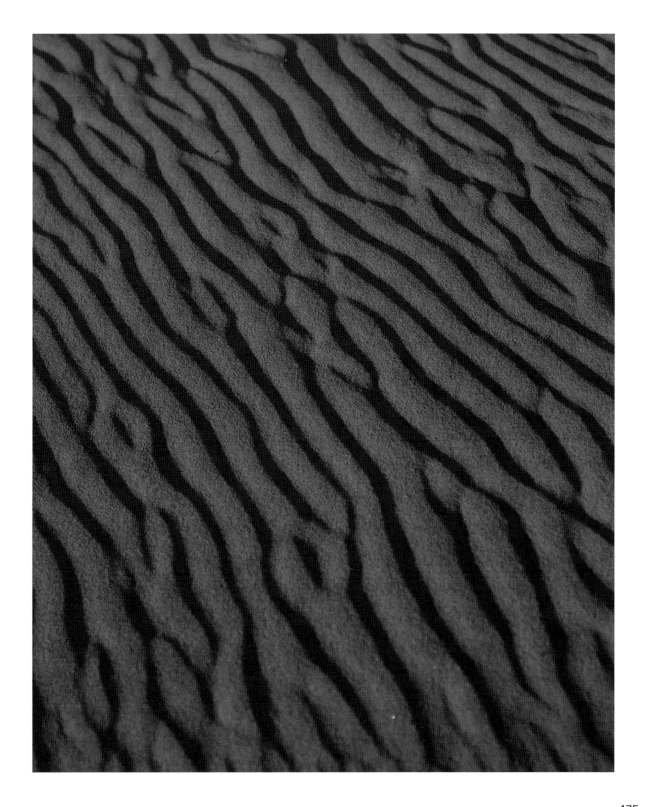

A LIFE OF MANY DEATHS

We will all experience the death of loved ones in our lives, and this will likely always be painful, no matter how much we have got in touch with the simple fact of mortality. But we ourselves go through a series of mini-deaths of our own, as we grow and evolve. A lot of the time, we're not aware of these deaths as they're happening. But we all move through childhood to adolescence, from our ambitious and energetic twenties, to our more settled and nurturing middle age, and into our older years. Each of these transitions involves the death of the person we once were. But even within these transitions, we will experience other mini-deaths. Perhaps the person who used to drink too much or comfort eat will die, making way for a healthier version. Perhaps the person who would allow themselves to be pushed around and exploited will make way for someone stronger with better boundaries. Perhaps the person who was a little selfish or cruel will make way for someone kinder and more empathetic.

In addition, certain experiences and rituals we once took part in and perhaps took for granted, will also end and die. There will be a last time you read your child a bedtime story with them snuggled up alongside you. There will be a last time you give your mother a hug. There will be a last time you kiss your partner. But you won't know it was the last time until after the event. Had you known beforehand, perhaps you would have taken your time and relished the experience a little bit more.

As we get older, we sometimes find ourselves looking back on our lives with a sense of loss. But none of us can live in the past, no matter how much we might want to. What matters is the present, and the path to the future we are creating. Rather than mourning who we used to be, we should celebrate the fact that we are evolving. These are positive deaths. And if we are truly thriving, we can expect to die positive deaths over and over again.

REGRETS OF THE DYING

Our reluctance to acknowledge mortality results in us taking each day for granted, not prioritizing our relationships, working too hard and pushing to achieve goals that won't actually make us happy. Bronnie Ware, the palliative care nurse and author of the bestseller *The Top Five Regrets of the Dying*, writes about the five most common regrets she heard from people at the end of their lives:

"I wish I'd had the courage to live a life true to myself, not the life others expected of me."

"I wish I hadn't worked so hard."

"I wish I'd had the courage to express my feelings."

"I wish I'd stayed in touch with my friends."

"I wish I'd let myself be happier."

Sitting beneath all of these regrets is a belief that life is an escalator and that there is infinite time to get things right. But there is not. Time is ticking, from the moment you are born.

I honestly believe that you dramatically reduce your chances of having these end-of-life regrets by accepting that you will die. It is death that brings life into sharp focus. Life is fragile. Life is finite. The fact that we are going to die is liberating and should be celebrated.

▶ **You can listen to the beautiful conversation I had with Bronnie Ware about the top regrets of the dying on Episode 383 of my *Feel Better, Live More* podcast at drchatterjee.com/383.**

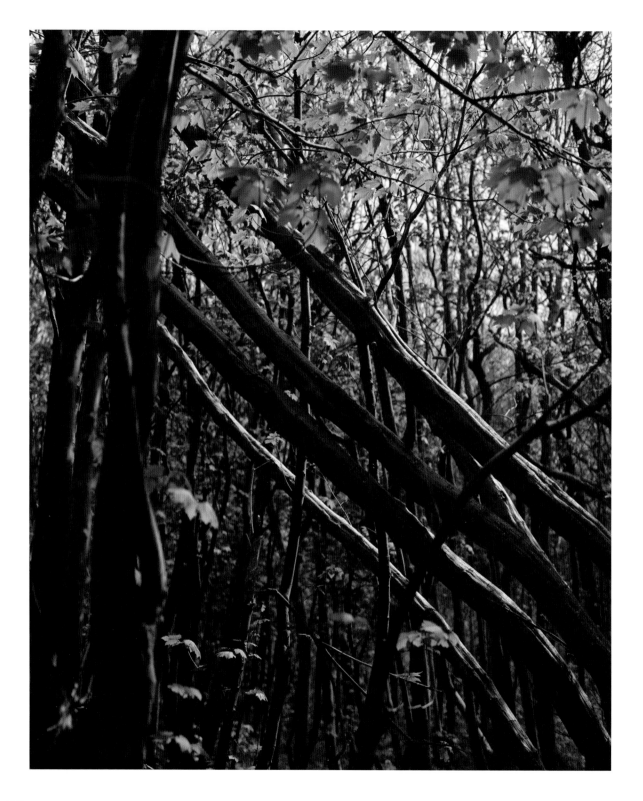

CONCLUSION

▶ Progress is nonlinear. When we rely on the idea that things will never go wrong in our lives, we set ourselves up for stress and failure. Life is not an escalator, it is an unpredictable landscape of peaks, troughs and long, meandering paths through the wilderness.

▶ When we sever the reliance on things never going wrong, we factor in inevitable temporary periods of stress and adversity. We realize that these periods are not signs that the world is out to get us. Rather than having a victim mindset, our mindset becomes that of a victor.

▶ The victim mindset is bad for us in many ways. It is poisonous to our mental and physical health. It makes us feel much less in control and creates emotional stress, which harms our minds and bodies. It also poisons our relationships because we become the kind of person who spends a lot of time complaining.

▶ The victim mindset also poisons our perception. It makes us blame everything bad that ever happens to us on the external world. Of course, sometimes other people will genuinely act unfairly and cause us difficulties. But it's always healthy to honestly interrogate the part we have played in our own problems, and ask what – if anything – we can do in the future to stop them happening again.

▶ The goal is to foster an outlook on life that is optimistic yet realistic. This includes the unavoidable fact that we will one day die.

▶ By learning to expect adversity, we deal with life's inevitable problems much more healthily. We will not be shocked when problems arrive. We will become more resilient, more positive and less reliant on the external world. This will make us immeasurably happier and healthier.

7. LET GO AND MOVE ON

Reliance on the past

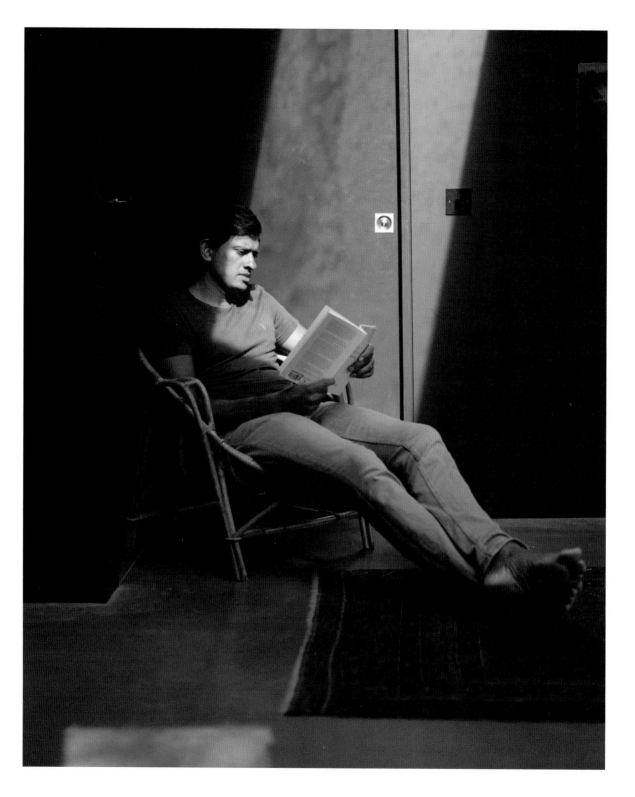

The patient who probably caused me the most personal upset, during my career as a GP, was a mother of three who I'll call Michelle. Michelle was a loving, wonderful person, a great mum and someone who was always fastidious about keeping herself fit and healthy. She maintained a strict wholefood diet with minimal alcohol or added sugar, swam and ran regularly, and walked her beloved dog Charlie twice a day. But, despite being physically well and comfortably off, Michelle found it impossible to thrive.

When she was just twenty-two, she discovered that her first husband had been having a long-term affair. After she confronted him about his betrayal he walked out, abandoning her and their young son. Michelle was never able to let go of this undeniably horrible event. Twenty-five years later, now in her mid-forties, she was still holding on to much of her resentment, frustration and anger. She remained so caught up in it all that her friends and family knew they couldn't say his name in front of her. In the end, despite my best efforts, I wasn't able to help Michelle. I urged her many times to try therapy or meditation to deal with her issues and help her move on, but she equated doing so with "forgiving" him for his affair, which she didn't want to do.

Sadly, Michelle ended up dying from cancer. My time treating her, coupled with a growing body of scientific research, got me thinking that, perhaps, the fact that she was unable to let go and move on from her past, played a role in her illness. There is an abundance of scientific literature supporting a strong link between unprocessed emotions and the development of a variety of chronic conditions. One study from Harvard found that women who have severe post-traumatic stress disorder have double the risk of developing ovarian cancer compared to women who don't. Another found that newly diagnosed people with colorectal cancer were more likely to demonstrate traits such as repression of anger, people-pleasing and the avoidance of conflict. Importantly, in this study, these personality traits and their association with cancer were independent of other well-established risk factors, such as family history, diet and alcohol intake. There is also evidence that people who hold on to anger and struggle to forgive have higher rates of autoimmune diseases, such as rheumatoid arthritis and lupus, compared to those who don't.

While none of these individual studies prove conclusively that unprocessed emotions directly cause these chronic diseases, if we take them alongside the observations of many experienced clinicians, it seems highly likely that at the very least, they play some role, alongside many other established factors, such as diet, alcohol, smoking, environmental toxin exposure, poverty, chronic stress and genetics. This highlights an important point that is often overlooked when we think about any chronic disease: in almost every single case, there are multiple factors that play a role in its development. It is exceptionally rare for only one factor to be the sole cause.

I want to make it abundantly clear that none of this is about blame. As we learned in Chapter 3, many of our behavioral traits, such as the tendency to people-please or repress our emotions, develop in childhood as necessary adaptations to ensure our basic needs get met. These traits served us exceptionally well when navigating the emotional environment of our early years but often become redundant, unhelpful and potentially harmful as we go about our lives as adults. We didn't consciously choose these patterns, so there is absolutely no reason for us to blame ourselves or feel guilty.

My intention in sharing this information is simply to help people realize that learning to let go of the past and move on is an important skill to cultivate in our quest for optimal health. As we've explored elsewhere, the mind and the body are massively interconnected. That interconnected system responds to the signals it receives from the world around us, and also from the world inside us. When we remain focused on past traumas, we tell our subconscious that the worst events that ever happened to us are still an active threat. We tell it that we are defined by those events, and our wellbeing is chained to them for ever. It hardly needs pointing out that, under these conditions, it's simply not possible to thrive.

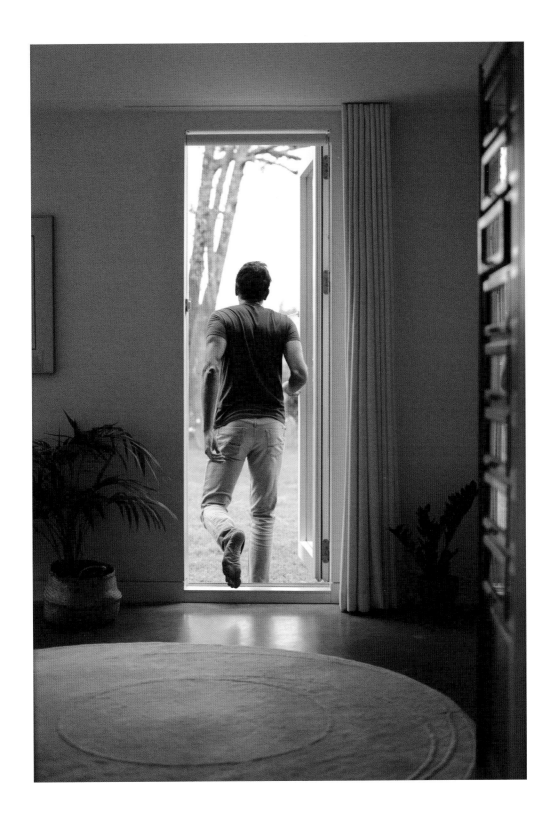

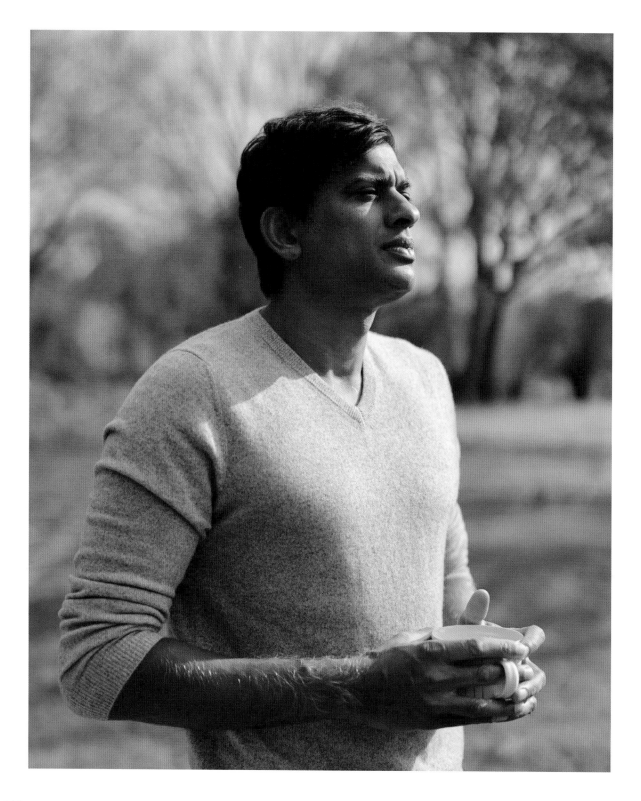

YOU ARE NOT YOUR PAST

I believe that many of us come to rely on our tales of trauma. This idea might seem strange – it might even lead you to feel a bit angry and defensive. Surely traumas are entirely negative events that most of us would do almost anything to erase? While this is true, it's also important to understand the ways that stories about our past can actually be helpful to us on a subconscious level.

Since the days of the inventor of psychotherapy, Sigmund Freud, we have become well used to looking backwards to incidents from our childhood to understand who we are in the present. This is completely valid. Talking therapies can be hugely beneficial to some people, and I'd never want to diminish them. There's no doubt in my mind that locating the source of our behavioral patterns and triggers can help us understand and unravel them.

But it's also true that, if we're not careful, we can use such stories as crutches. Everyone has something about them that is fragile or damaged, or has been unfairly judged as "not good enough" by other people. Perhaps you've suffered from a serious illness, have a disability, had abusive or alcoholic parents, or have suffered dependency yourself. Maybe you were raised in poverty, suffered from bullying or experienced some form of discrimination. Perhaps, like Michelle, you have had bitter misfortune in love. Whatever your "held-back" narrative is, I've no doubt it is true and real and the source of utterly justified pain and anger to you. My question for you is not whether it's real, but whether you've become reliant on it.

When we overly identify with our harm narrative, we invite pity. Like sugar, or any number of even more addictive drugs, pity can feel good in the moment but more than a very modest dose of it is toxic. When we repeat our harm narrative, we send a message out to the world, and into our subconscious brains, that we believe special allowances should be made for us. How can we be expected to move on when we have suffered so much? How can we be expected to push ourselves, and try just that little bit harder to improve our lives, when we have been so hard done by?

Michelle wasn't able to face the emotional discomfort of forgiving her first husband. Rather than saying "my problem is my inability to move on," she told herself, "my problem is that I've been dreadfully wronged by this horrible man." This story generated pity from other people. It also generated a huge amount of self-pity. The story felt comforting to her and gave her permission not to change. This is how she came to rely on it. And by doing so, she allowed herself to be defined by the very worst thing that had ever happened to her and gave away all her power to the man she hated. Again, I want to emphasize that none of this is about blame or judgement. I understand that moving on from difficult past experiences can be challenging but I want to assure you that doing so is always worth it.

For many of us, the past becomes our safe space. Even if it contains episodes of serious trauma, we are afraid to leave it behind. It's easier to stay with what we know. Letting go of the past means taking on new feelings and becoming a new person – and that can be frightening. But that fright, which is perfectly natural and understandable, can keep us relying on the past. It stops us from growing, because growth only happens when we get outside our comfort zone.

STORIES THAT LIMIT US

It's hard to overstate the power that stories have to hold us back. Up until 1954 nobody had ever run a mile in four minutes or less. Most athletes simply didn't believe this feat was possible. The four-minute mile was finally cracked by the British runner Roger Bannister, and guess what happened next? Runners all over the world began busting through this once impenetrable boundary. Today, well over 1,600 athletes around the globe have run four-minute miles. Human physiology couldn't possibly have evolved so rapidly. So what changed? The point is that Roger Bannister didn't just break a record back in 1954, he also broke a story that the wider running world believed, one that had been holding them back. People suddenly realized the feat could be achieved, and it became true. What this tells me is that we can never achieve anything unless we believe it is possible.

"We can never achieve anything unless we believe it is possible."

YOU ARE NOT YOUR ILLNESS

It's not only harm narratives from the past that can become reliances that prevent personal growth. As unlikely as it might seem, patients suffering from chronic illness can unknowingly become overly identified with their condition, which can help prevent them from getting better. In the second series of the BBC documentary that I made, *Doctor in the House*, I treated a woman who had a ten-year history of chronic pain, which had been diagnosed as fibromyalgia. Nicola's life was awful. She had to sleep a lot during the day, she couldn't be the mum she wanted to be to her kids and she couldn't work – she couldn't even walk around the block, let alone manage a daily commute.

The day I started working with Nicola, I discovered that the BBC had arranged for her to have an appointment with one of the top pain specialists in London, in four weeks' time. When I asked why they had done this, they said they thought it would help her manage her pain better. I told them, "Guys, I don't want to help her manage her pain. I want to get her out of pain completely." They asked how I could possibly do that. "I don't know yet," I said. "Let me get to know her and I'll try my best to figure it out. In the meantime, I want you to cancel that appointment."

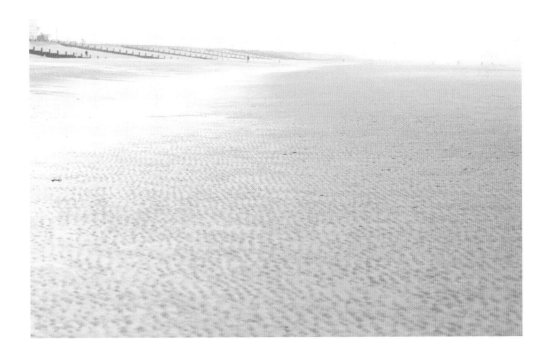

Six weeks later Nicola was completely pain free for the first time in ten years, without the use of any medication. It was one of the proudest achievements of my life. When the episode went out, I was excited about the response we'd get. Immediately after the broadcast there were thousands of positive comments online. But, to my shock, what I also saw was a barrage of abuse. People were saying all kinds of negative things about me, criticizing my approach and alleging that Nicola never had fibromyalgia in the first place. I found this extremely hard to deal with. Vidh and I were so upset we didn't sleep for several nights. We couldn't understand it. Why was I being attacked? I hadn't used any medication; instead I'd shown her how to become pain free by helping her make small but significant tweaks to her lifestyle and by helping her change the way she viewed herself and the world around her. How could this possibly be seen as a bad thing?

But then I began to see a clear pattern in my online attackers. Many of them had Twitter tags like "FibroDavid," "FibroJane," and "FibroTash." That's when it clicked. These were people whose entire identities had been swallowed up by their diagnoses. I immediately started to feel compassion for them. I realized they were struggling so much with their own health issues that it was just too much for them to accept what I'd helped Nicola do. Her release from pain, in many ways, invalidated their struggle, and their struggle had become who they were. They were stuck in their illnesses. The belief that they might actually be able to recover, after so many years of pain, as well as – perhaps – feeling invalidated by their doctors, was like an insult to them. It diminished the story they told themselves about who they were.

YOU ARE A MORNING PERSON

In some cases, it's not a harm narrative that has become an invisible crutch, but a limiting idea from our past that has somehow stuck to us. One of my patients was a single dad who was always stressed and suffered with from high blood pressure. He confessed he'd often be reactive towards his children over breakfast and then behind the wheel of his car on the school run. He'd get out of bed every morning at 7:45. When I asked him if it would not be better for him to set his alarm a bit earlier, he told me, "No chance. I'm not a morning person. Never have been, not since I was a teenager." I wondered where he'd picked up this story. It seemed obvious to me that it was an invisible reliance that was holding him back. I explained to him that, although some of us do have genetic tendencies to be either a morning or an evening person, the reality is that our body clocks can often be shifted depending on how we live our lives. I have seen a "night owl" becoming a "morning lark" and vice versa. He told me he'd try a short period of setting the alarm for 6 a.m. and turning off his screens ninety minutes earlier each evening. To his amazement, after a couple of weeks, he was falling asleep ninety minutes earlier and rising in good time without an issue. This modest change to his routine resulted in his blood pressure coming down and his feeling less stressed and much calmer – which was no doubt greatly appreciated by his two sons.

START WITH ZERO:
HOW THE PAST HAUNTS
OUR RELATIONSHIPS

So much of the conflict we experience in our personal relationships comes as a result of us bringing stories and ideas from the past into the present. We allow prior experiences to color our present-day interactions, making assumptions about another's behavior or motivations based on problems we've encountered previously.

I've recently been experimenting with an approach in my own life that I think of as "starting with zero." I've challenged myself to show up in every interaction with my wife Vidh as if it was the first time. Can I experience the present interaction with her in the moment, without bringing in preconceived ideas from the past?

I'll be honest, I haven't found it easy. After all, we're actually working against our minds when we do this; our brains work by constantly trying to predict the future based on our past experiences. But the amazing thing about our brains is that we can literally rewire them. We can free ourselves from our pasts if we choose to.

▶ Could you adopt a "starting with zero" approach with someone in your own life? Perhaps for seven days? Pay close attention to how things feel when you are trying this out compared to when you don't.

Every time I mindfully adopt a "start from zero" approach with Vidh, I feel I am creating a different relationship with her. I feel lighter, freer and more present with her as we talk. And, almost immediately, this gets reciprocated back. The more intentional effort I put into starting with zero, the easier and more instinctive it becomes.

If you try this approach with someone in your life, almost certainly, you will quickly realize how many of your present-day interactions are influenced by the past. Armed with that knowledge, you can start to change things going forward.

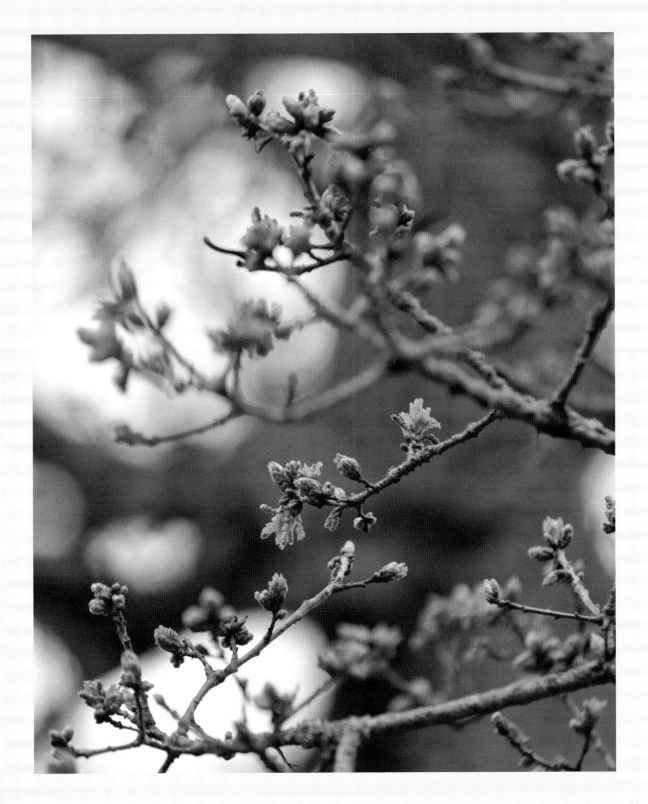

THE ASTONISHING POWER OF FORGIVENESS

If you have any remaining doubts about how damaging our reliance on past stories can be, I hope you will be convinced by what scientists have found happens when we cultivate the skill of letting them go. Forgiveness of others has been shown to improve the quality of our relationships, lessen anxiety and stress, reduce blood pressure, improve our immune system function and help with self-esteem.

Dr. Fred Luskin from Stanford University is one of the world's leading forgiveness researchers. He describes forgiveness as the "peace and understanding that comes from lessening the blame of that which has hurt you, taking your life experience less personally and seeing the cost of holding a grudge." He describes three types of forgiveness: interpersonal, intrapersonal and existential. Interpersonal forgiveness involves letting go of an offense we perceive someone else to have committed against us. Intrapersonal forgiveness is about forgiving ourselves for something we have previously done. Existential forgiveness is about forgiving the universe or nature or God for what we perceive them to have done to us.

Research on the power of forgiveness is clear. Love will pay you back in a way that hate never will. But it's not always easy. Just as my former patient Michelle experienced, forgiveness can be hard because it feels like we're doing a huge favor to someone who has hurt us. But forgiveness is not about freeing people from blame for the things they've done to us. It's about freeing ourselves from their damage. When we forgive, the only person we're granting a favor to is us. As Desmond Tutu once said, "without forgiveness there is no future." When we don't forgive, we lock ourselves in the past. Only we can turn the key and unlock the doorway to a future of thriving.

Forgiveness becomes easier when we approach it with the right mindset. We make it much harder on ourselves when we think: "That person wronged me, yet I need to push through and forgive." Forgiveness that is underpinned by a conscious feeling of resistance is destined to fail. It has an energy state that means we are

▶ **To listen to the incredible conversation I had with Fred Luskin go to Episode 448 of my** *Feel Better, Live More* **podcast at drchatterjee.com/448.**

actively trying to "overcome" something, rather than go with its flow. As a general rule of life, whenever we try to overcome rather than flow with, we run into problems.

If you try to forgive from a place of judgement, you will find it difficult. But coming from a place of compassion and acceptance makes forgiveness come effortlessly. If you choose to believe that everyone is doing the best that they can, given their unique circumstances – their childhood, their parents, their life experiences – and weaknesses, and that we all inevitably get things wrong and make mistakes, you quickly realize there is nothing to actively forgive. You move beyond it. Forgiveness happens naturally.

This type of approach really appeals to me as a doctor. I have always been fascinated with the root cause of my patients' problems, as opposed to having a myopic focus on their symptoms. Problems like back pain and headaches usually have upstream causes, which often means just treating the head or the back is a mistake. This is also a valuable way of approaching forgiveness. Pull the right upstream lever, and forgiveness occurs as a natural by-product. And the upstream lever is simple: acceptance and compassion.

This is true when it comes to forgiving others, and it's also true when forgiving ourselves. When we have regrets or beat ourselves up over things we've done, we don't think about the fact that it was an older, less wise version of ourselves that was doing the best they could with what they knew at the time. This even holds true if we're regretting something we did yesterday or even an hour ago, and we should have more compassion than to beat ourselves up in our own minds. When we're not able to forgive ourselves, we risk becoming paralyzed with shame, guilt and regret. This generates a huge amount of internal stress, damages our self-worth and makes it much more likely we'll engage in unhealthy behaviors. As a consequence, we feel stuck in our lives and find it challenging to make positive changes.

I've come to believe that regret is a form of perfectionism. At its core is the belief that we have the capability to be perfect and make perfect decisions, and the fact that we didn't means that we've somehow failed. But the truth is that all of us are imperfect and when we do make mistakes those mistakes are usually not apparent

Note: If you want to try out some of my practical exercises on forgiveness, please take a look at my third book, *Feel Better in 5,* or visit drchatterjee.com/forgiveness.

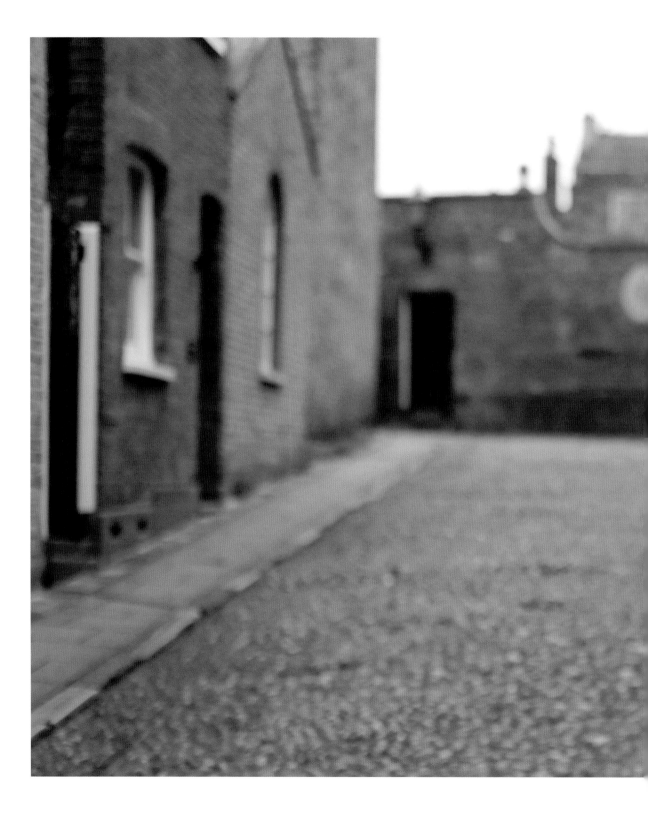

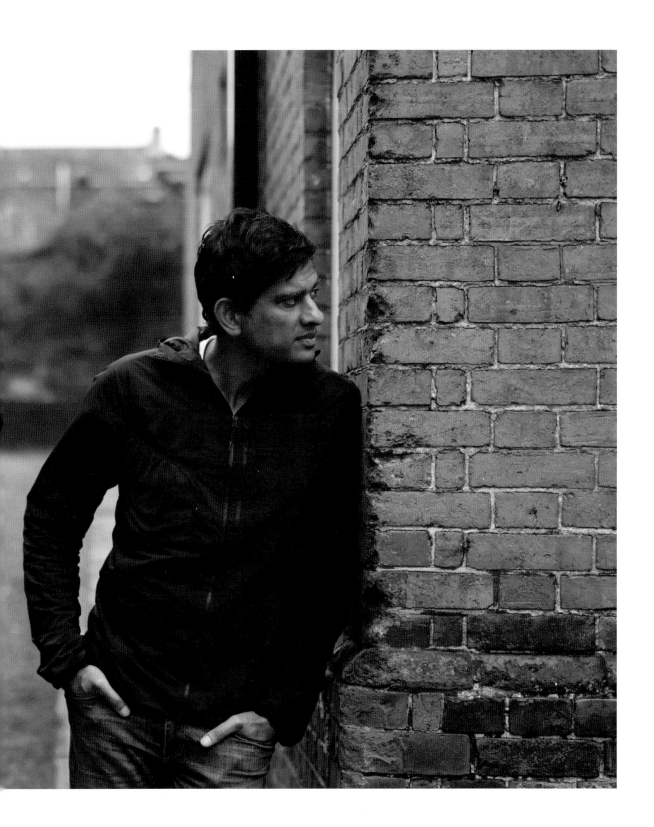

until sometime after. That doesn't mean we can't learn from the past and make better decisions going forward. Of course, we can. But it really doesn't help us to look back on our past mistakes with negativity and guilt. It's much better if we can be compassionate to ourselves and accept that we made certain choices in the past which had certain consequences and, if faced with similar situations again, we'll choose to make different ones. If we could have done better, we would have done. And, now that we do, we will.

CAN YOU FORGIVE YOURSELF?

When he was just five years old, the former American football player Lewis Howes was raped by the son of his babysitter. He didn't tell a soul until he was thirty-one years old. The anger and shame locked up inside him, over all those years, made him reactive, angry and unpredictable. He was forty-one when I spoke to him on my podcast and he told me, "I had to learn how to forgive him." But he also needed to forgive himself. He realized that for years he'd been beating himself up with shame and abusing himself emotionally and mentally. "I had to forgive myself for the twenty-five years of pain that I had caused me," he said.

This insight from Lewis absolutely stopped me in my tracks. I found it so profound. Yes, the rape happened. It shouldn't have and it was in no way his fault. But what he realized was that *he* was the one who allowed the pain to continue all those years, which meant only *he* could do something about it. I think we can all learn so much from Lewis's hard-won wisdom. Many of us torture ourselves about things that happened months and years ago. But if we keep on living in the past, we lose our present. We allow yesterday to sabotage today.

▶ **To listen to my full conversation with Lewis Howes, go to Episode 346 of my *Feel Better, Live More* podcast at drchatterjee.com/346.**

CHANGE YOUR MEMORY, CHANGE YOUR PAST

One reason we find ourselves tied to things that happened long ago is that our pasts live on inside us, in the form of memories. Often these memories are extremely painful and can feel impossible to let go. But it is possible to change and heal them. I have done exactly this during Internal Family Systems therapy sessions (see Chapter 3). In one particular session, I remembered something that happened when I was eight years old. Under the guidance of my therapist, I went back to that event in my memory as my forty-year-old self and made peace with it. I talked to my eight-year-old self, telling him I understand how he feels and that I care and will always be there for him, and then I helped him take a different perspective on the situation. Remarkably, I have found that after these sessions, I respond differently to situations that previously would have triggered me. This is because, when I was being triggered, it was that wounded eight-year-old that lived on in me that was crying out in pain. Revisiting the memory healed him, and healed me.

When I spoke to the world-renowned sleep expert Professor Matthew Walker about this on my podcast, he explained that scientists have indeed found that memories are changeable. The phase of sleep called REM is thought to be a form of "emotional first aid." You can think of it as a type of therapeutic process the brain carries out on itself. It involves taking the hard edges off our painful experiences, so they get stored with less of an emotional charge. So, day to day, as long as we are sleeping well, our brains are trying to help us by reducing the impact of negative events. However, Professor Walker explained to me that you can actually go back in and update or "change" a memory. "Every time you recall the memory, you open it back up to the possibility of change," he told me. "You can change its content, you can update it and you can modify it. Potentially, you can even remove some parts of it, but you can also update the context and the emotional tenor of that memory – and then you go and press the save button." Technically this process is called reconsolidation. It is proof that we are not prisoners of our past and that, with a bit of work, we can even alter memories that have been holding us back and preventing us from thriving.

▶ **To listen to the conversation I had with Matthew Walker, go to Episode 147 of my *Feel Better, Live More* podcast at drchatterjee.com/147.**

PRACTICE, REHEARSE, VISUALIZE

Top sports stars and CEOs have a valuable practice that truly helps free them from the past. Many report that visualizing who they want to become in the future can have a transformative effect on their lives, and helps them achieve optimal performance.

Ed Moses, one of the greatest hurdlers of all time, was known to lie with his eyes closed next to one of the hurdles on the track while his fellow competitors were warming up. He imagined the starter's gun going off, the sensation of his legs driving out of the block, the feel of the grip of his spikes against the track, the sensation of his trail leg coming smoothly over the hurdles and every one of the thirteen steps he would take between every hurdle. Between 1977 and 1987, Moses won 107 consecutive finals. This a truly exceptional and unsurpassed feat and he believes visualization played a crucial part in it.

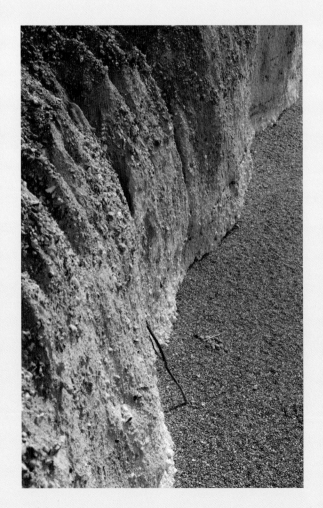

Visualization has also been found to help people who have suffered a stroke. Precise visualization of their weaker side doing certain activities, like picking up a glass of water, makes them recover faster. There are even studies that show just imagining the eating of food can reduce how much we want to eat afterward.

The great thing about visualization is that it really doesn't need to take that long. Every day, towards the end of my own morning routine, I ask myself a series of questions that help me visualize the kind of person I wish to be

▶ How do I want to act today?

▶ How do I want to show up with my wife?

▶ How do I want to interact with the people I work with?

▶ What are past behaviors of mine that I no longer wish to repeat?

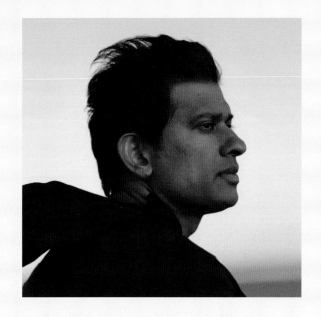

I finish off this exercise by writing down in my journal the answer to one all-encompassing question:

▶ Which quality or qualities do I want to showcase to the world today?

Just by becoming conscious of your previous behaviors that you no longer wish to embody, and writing down the quality you wish to showcase to the world, you prime your brain to be a better person each day. You are much more likely to behave in the way you want if you have spent a few moments intentionally thinking about it.

I recommend writing the answers down in a journal. This forces you to take a pause and properly articulate your thoughts. If you have the time, you can also imagine with all of your senses what it would feel like to showcase that

quality. You could spend a few moments visualizing how you want to be when you go into that meeting with your boss, first see your kids after school, or greet your partner after a day at work.

If you're not mentally practicing the new you, you'll be more likely to fall into old patterns. Your thoughts and actions will be predicated on the past. But you are not your past. You are not an inevitable result of who you used to be.

"Which quality or qualities do I want to showcase to the world today?"

LET IT GO

Bessel van der Kolk, the author of *The Body Keeps the Score*, told me on my podcast that the problem with trauma is not the actual event, but our reaction to it. Why are we reacting negatively to something that happened years ago? The past is over. It happened. The fact is, we have all had positive and negative experiences. If we focus on only the bad things that have happened to us, we keep ourselves trapped and tied to our pasts. It's simply not possible to thrive under circumstances like these.

But there is another path we can choose. The amazing thing is, when we make the positive decision to live as a lighter, freer person in the present, we rewrite our pasts. We make those ideas and incidents that held us back less powerful. Of course, I do understand that many of us have had extremely traumatic experiences that are very difficult to process. Letting go can be a long and difficult journey. But by killing the ghosts of yesterday, we free ourselves to thrive today.

▶ **To listen to my conversation with Bessel van der Kolk, go to Episode 336 of my *Feel Better, Live More* podcast at drchatterjee.com/336.**

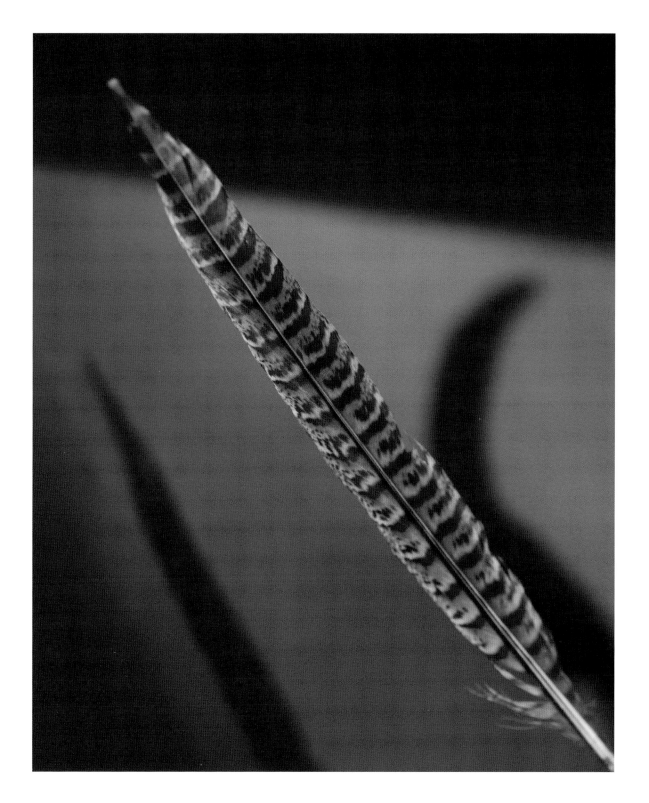

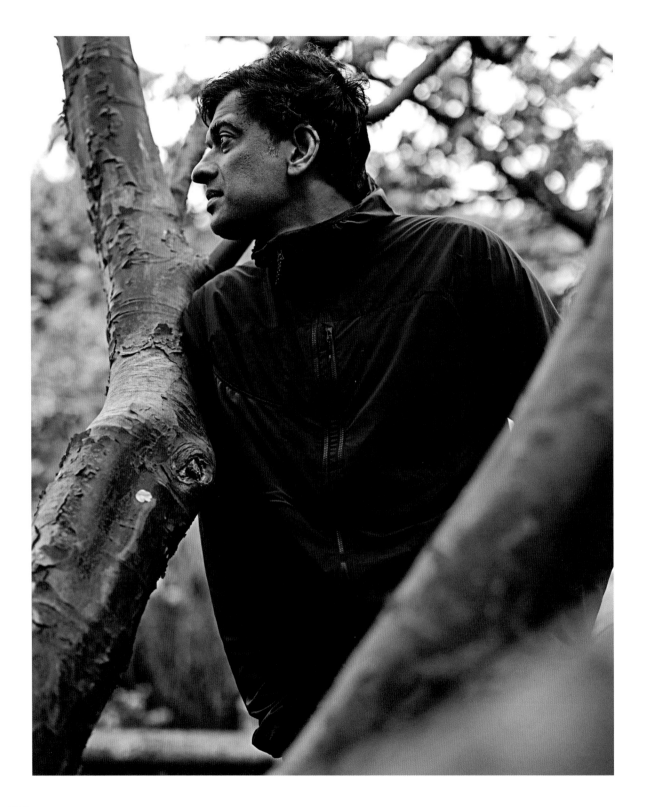

CONCLUSION

▶ Many of us become overly reliant on our past experiences. For some of us, they become a source of our identity and a reliance that we use to justify unhelpful behaviors. But holding on to pain and resentment not only causes anger, anxiety and depression; some research suggests a potential link with certain chronic diseases.

▶ Stories from our past can negatively impact our present relationships. To overcome this, we can practice "starting from zero" with every interaction we have with our loved ones. To start from zero is to meet our friends and family as if we're free of any baggage that has damaged our relationships in the past.

▶ Forgiveness is also a powerful tool for breaking our reliance on the past. It's important to remember that this is not about letting someone "get away" with what they did nor is it about saying that what happened was OK. It is about freeing yourself from the burden of the past and allowing yourself to fully experience the present. Forgiveness becomes much easier if you adopt a compassionate mindset. We also benefit from taking this approach with ourselves, who we also need to forgive for past experiences that have resulted in us feeling regret, shame or guilt.

▶ We can move on from our pasts by revisiting and rewriting painful memories. Of course, this may sometimes require the help of a therapist. We can also try visualizing who we want to become in the future, a practice employed successfully by many top sports stars and CEOs. By cutting our reliance on our past, we make a positive decision to live as a lighter, freer person in the present – and the future.

8. RECLAIM YOUR TIME

Reliance on busyness

If you had told me as a child that I'd one day have my own BBC Radio 2 show, my mind would have been blown. It would be like telling me that all my dreams were going to come true and that my adult life was going to be completely perfect. OK, so I didn't wind up being Jon Bon Jovi. But becoming a radio DJ was almost as epic. I wonder how that same child would feel on being told that, two years into this incredible job, I would decide to just get up and walk away from it?

I imagine I'd be both confused and furious. My younger self would be raging at middle-aged me, asking if I'd gone totally mad. But walk away is exactly what I did, in May 2022. There were a few reasons for this, but by far the most important was a question I asked myself as my mother's health deteriorated. I wondered, when she inevitably dies, was I going to look back on this period of my life and think, "I'm really glad I did all those extra hours of work and made my name as a BBC Radio DJ"? Or would I think, "I wish I'd spent more time with Mum when she'd been around"?

There's no question I'm pleased with my decision to quit. But the truth is, it wasn't an easy one to make. I went back and forth on it for many months and agonized during semi-sleepless nights. What I have accepted now is that I should never have really taken the job in the first place. I spent two years struggling to find the bandwidth to do it. It resulted in a great deal of stress and stole me away from parts of my life that were much more important, not least my family and friends. I really didn't have the time for the show, and yet I thought I could somehow squash it into my already packed calendar.

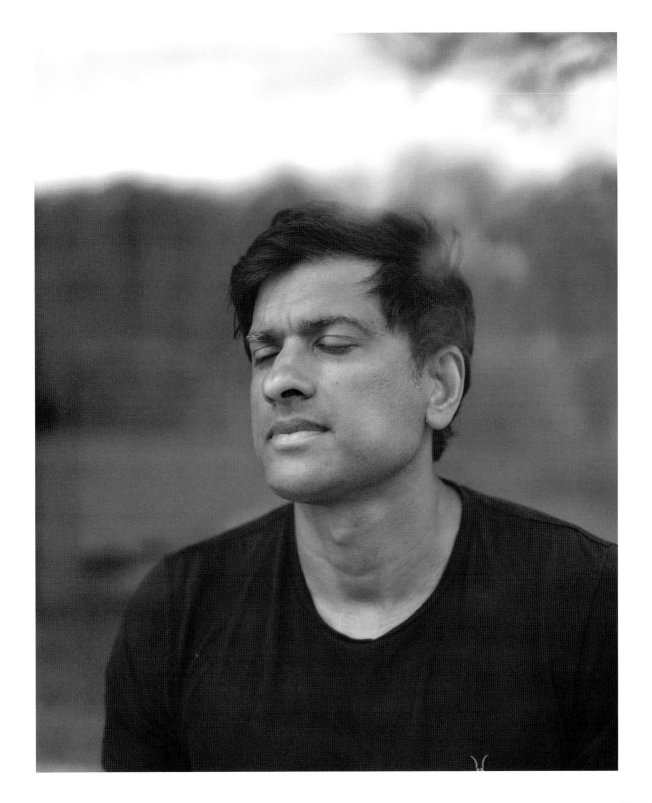

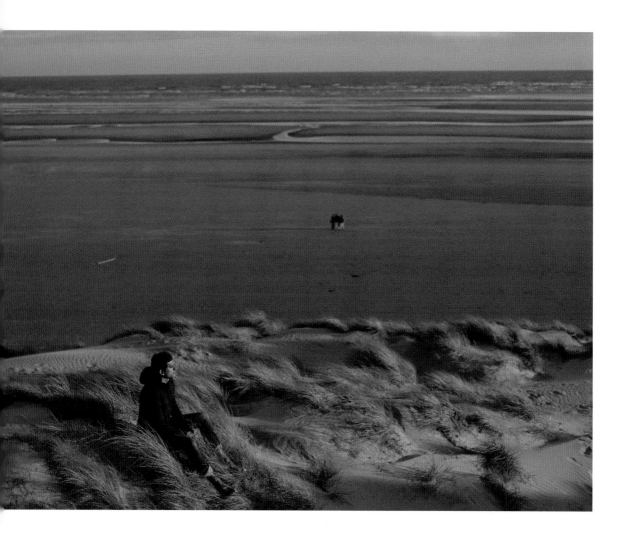

When I ask myself why I said yes in the first place, the answer is simple. Because I still have that excited little boy inside me, and that little boy equated having my own national radio show with success. So what if it made me crazily busy? When I was that kid, dreaming of my future as a successful adult, busyness was exactly what I pictured. I grew up watching Hollywood movies that opened on helicopter shots of New York skyscrapers and then zoomed into the hero or heroine in sharp business clothes, striding up the sidewalk with their briefcase and a mobile phone the length of a size thirteen shoe, moving through a sea of other smart, ambitious commuters at the start of another nonstop day. In a society that's still very much focused on money and status, we have images like these drummed into us from an early age: to thrive is to be busy. Busyness and success are one and the same.

But this is a terrible lesson to teach our children. Because, make no mistake, it is a myth. And it's no exaggeration to say that this myth is killing us. Millions of us have absorbed the idea that we can only be successful if we are constantly busy. And this affliction doesn't only affect the young and ambitious: I know grandmothers who have spent their lives raising children and struggle to sit still in their eighties, never having learned the simple and underrated pleasure of doing nothing. We feel that if we are not constantly busy, we are somehow failing at life. In fact the opposite is true: it is constant busyness that will make our lives fail and prevent us from thriving.

BUSYNESS IS LAZINESS

Rather than being a sign of success, busyness can often be a sign of laziness. For many of us, it signals that we haven't organized our life properly and are too focused on one aspect of it at the expense of all others. Of course, some of us can't help being incredibly busy. Perhaps we are a single parent struggling to pay our bills and bring up our kids. Perhaps we are a mother or father who is trying to run a business, spend time with our children and care for elderly parents without much support. There are times in our life when busyness seems to be the only option. But the truth is that lots of us – dare I say most of us – are a lot busier than we actually need to be.

Reducing our state of busyness means allowing ourselves to prioritize the things we have to do, and learning to say no to the things that are pushing us over our stress thresholds. It begins with accepting the basic fact that we will never have time to do everything that is asked of us. There are only so many hours in a day, and we can only be awake and functioning properly for around sixteen of them. Without thinking, we sometimes act as if we will find happiness and peace only when we get to the end of our list of jobs and responsibilities. But there is no end to that list. There will always be something else that our bosses, partners or children would like us to do. There will always be jobs to be done around the house. The to-do list of an ordinary adult is like a magic bucket that keeps refilling itself forever. We will never thrive unless we accept this truth, learn to prioritize and learn to say no.

Saying no to things we don't want to do often means risking upsetting people, which means they might like us less (a reliance I cover in detail in Chapter 3). But we also need to get used to saying no to things we do want to do, which is difficult for other reasons. Nevertheless, we have to be strong enough to make hard choices.

We have to get used to making sacrifices. I myself can be a bit of a dreamer. I want to be a surfer, an elite marathon runner, a great swimmer, a musician and a songwriter. I want to learn martial arts and at least three new languages. (I am not exaggerating. I really do want all of these things!) But over the past few years I have had to admit to myself that there is simply no way I can achieve all those things and have the life I truly want. Pursuing these goals would mean I would not be able to be an attentive husband, a responsible father, a well-prepared podcast host and a good friend to the people I love. So, I have had to make hard choices. I have had to put limitations on my life. But with these limitations comes freedom.

BUSYNESS AND THE ETERNAL QUEST FOR STATUS

I recently had a conversation with Will Storr, the author of a book called *The Status Game*, on my podcast. He told me about recent scientific research that has found status to be a universal driver in humans. It turns out that we all seek it, even if unconsciously. Contrary to what you might assume, seeking status doesn't necessarily mean chasing wealth or celebrity or high-powered jobs. It's simply the feeling that we're offering value to the world around us. All of us want to believe that other people think we're good at something, whether this judgement is related to our work lives or hobbies. Even being a good Christian, a good Buddhist or a good mother or father counts.

The seeking of status should not necessarily be seen as a bad thing. Back in the hunter-gatherer tribes we evolved in, we would have received status for being a great forager of sweet potatoes or a successful hunter or wonderful storyteller. The problem is, in today's culture, we award status for behaviors and activities that aren't always good for us. On top of that, many of us view busy people as having more status because we perceive them as being capable, ambitious and in demand.

Over the past few years, I have come to believe that our reliance on busyness comes from a fear of insignificance. Because our lives now are so disconnected and individualistic, busyness helps us feel important. When I look at cultures around the world that are happier than ours, and have relatively high rates of longevity, one thing that stands out to me is that their lives are full of meaning. They know deeply that they are of value to the people around them. In the West, we are becoming more and more disconnected, living away from our tribes, families and networks – often in the pursuit of a better job or an enticing opportunity. This creates a deep unconscious fear that we are not of value. This is why we are all hell-bent on trying to prove we have status by always appearing busy.

We can also fall into the trap of obsessing over our children's status. It's completely natural for kids – and especially adolescents – to be concerned about where they sit in the social pecking order. But I often see parents actively encouraging this kind of thinking. They often over-schedule their children in an attempt to keep up with the Joneses. I know of a popular swimming club and often hear mums and dads praising it, remarking on how it has helped their kids rapidly improve their skills. I have no doubt that this is true. But the pay-off is that their kids are also having repeated early mornings and late nights during the week, leading to physical and emotional exhaustion. They will often break down in tears due to the huge amount of extra pressure that's put on them. Is this success? Is your child becoming a better swimmer worth it if the cost is exhaustion, despair and low self-worth?

If this is an easy trap to fall into, it is because of how the brain is wired. In my previous book *Happy Mind, Happy Life* I describe how the brain's "system of desire" fools us into thinking things like status are the key to happiness. My dad worked himself to an early grave because he was so convinced that his work would make him and those around him happy, that he spent thirty years sleeping just three nights a week. There are millions of people out there, just like my dad, who are making themselves ill by overprioritizing one aspect of their lives. For the last few years, a big part of my medical practice has been the treatment of patients with autoimmune disease. In at least 95 percent of cases, I've seen a high level of stress in a patient's life during the six months prior to the onset of symptoms. It would be radically oversimplifying things to say that stress is the simple and sole cause of their problem. But it does indicate how bad chronic, unmanaged stress is for us generally, and how it sets up the conditions for us to fall seriously ill.

It also interferes with our powers of insight. When we're busy, we're lost in a storm of stress signals from all the demands that are being made of us. That makes it almost impossible to make out what needs to be heard inside ourselves. As we learned in Chapter 1, when we lose the power of insight, it means we're more likely to deal with moments of stress by defaulting to our unhealthy habits.

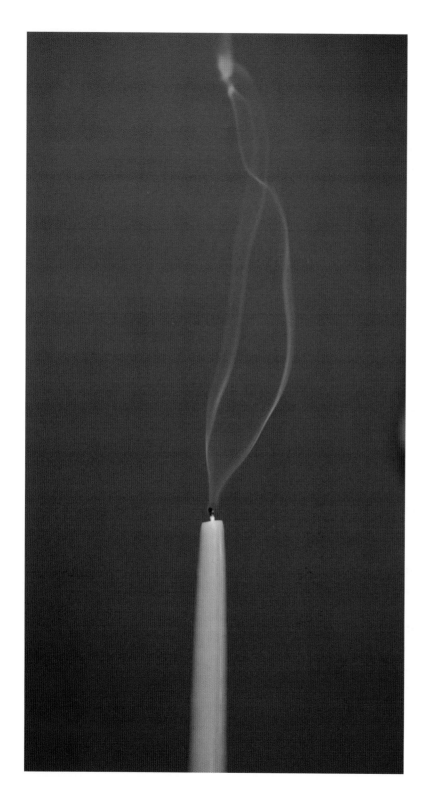

THE BURNOUT EPIDEMIC

I know from my GP work that our reliance on busyness is causing an epidemic of burnout. It is highly likely that you or someone close to you is right now on the road to this very real and damaging condition. One survey showed that 88 percent of UK workers had suffered from burnout in the past two years. I find this staggering. Whether this truly reflects the current situation across the entire UK, I am not so sure, but it is an alarming statistic that should demand we all sit up and take notice. What does it say about us as a society?

To understand what burnout is, picture a rubber band. If you pull a rubber band a little bit and then let it go, it happily returns to its original shape. This is how our stress response should work. A little bit of stress is totally fine and, in fact, often pushes us to perform at our best. If we give ourselves a sensible amount of time to recover from episodes of stress, we should happily return to normal. However, many of us keep pushing ourselves and pushing ourselves, day after day. We find ourselves checking emails late into the evening and during the weekends. We prioritize overtime above time with our loved ones and worry about work problems constantly. In other words, we fail to allow ourselves enough space to rest and recuperate.

Now imagine that rubber band again. If we keep pulling at it, day after day, week after week, beyond what its natural capability allows, it starts to deform. This is exactly what happens to our stress response when we experience burnout. We have pushed so hard and for so long, it starts to change shape. This change in shape alters how we feel and how we think. We turn into a different person. We become reactive and volatile, tired and wired. This is the reality for many of us these days. The shape of our stress response system is becoming deformed.

When I come across someone who describes themselves as a workaholic, I'll often ask them, "What's your endgame?" The fact is, if they continue to rely on busyness in order to feel happy, there's a high chance they will suffer from some form of burnout or a serious illness, or see their marriage break down, or have a difficult relationship with their children. Even if they do manage to dodge all these missiles, they are putting themselves in the line for a miserable retirement. If they haven't nourished all the parts of their lives that aren't focused on their careers, they may well find themselves facing a twilight of emptiness and depression.

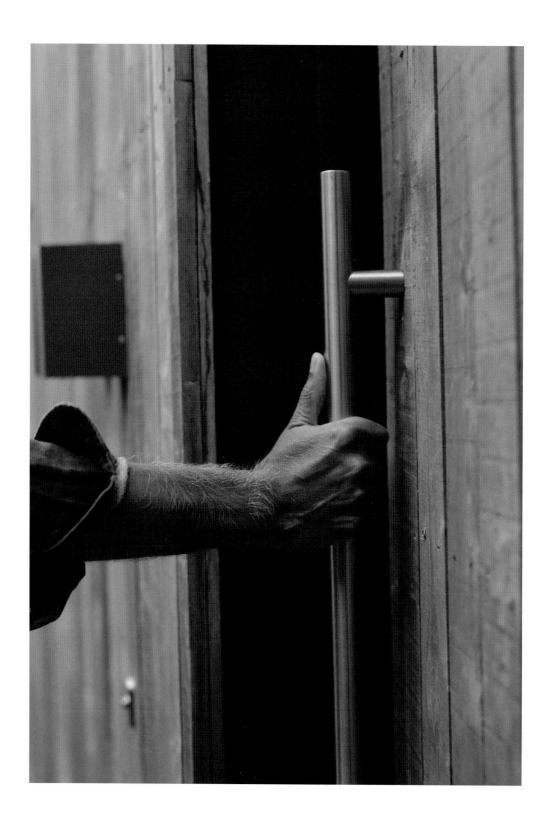

CASE STUDY

A few years ago, I treated a 55-year-old man named Ahmed who had developed the autoimmune disease, lupus. To suffer from any autoimmune illness, experts, like Dr. Alessio Fasano from Harvard, believe that three conditions need to be met. A person needs to be genetically susceptible, suffer from increased intestinal permeability (colloquially known as leaky gut) and exposed to some sort of environmental trigger, such as chronic, unmanaged stress. Ahmed had a family history of autoimmune disease, so quite possibly had the genetic predisposition. Some of his symptoms suggested that he may have an issue with increased intestinal permeability. But, without an environmental trigger (chronic stress), he potentially would never have developed the illness.

Ahmed owned a minicab company and would work incessantly, often late into the night. He already had enough income to live comfortably. But he kept pushing and working long hours, telling himself that this was just for a few more years until he had just a little bit more. Ultimately, his lupus forced him to give up his work and sell his business. It's impossible to say for sure that overwork is what caused his illness, but I have seen a similar pattern over and over again with many of my patients.

Contrast Ahmed's experience with that of a close friend of mine, who always seemed to have self-awareness beyond his years. In his early thirties, he was working as a high school teacher. He was offered a promotion to Head of History but turned it down, as he realized it would mean coming home later from school in the evenings, working every weekend, and spending less time with his family. Fifteen years on, that friend of mine is thriving. He still enjoys his job, but crucially he has time to pursue his passions and spends lots of quality time with his family.

From what I have seen, this kind of self-awareness is pretty rare, especially in someone in their thirties. Far too many of us fall for the false cultural narrative that tells us more money and promotion is always better. When we fill our lives solely with our work, we make a trade. We swap our family, friends and physical and mental health for our careers. And the big question we all have to ask ourselves is this: are these trades we're making with our lives every day really worth it?

SIX SIGNS OF BURNOUT

The problem with burnout is that it is usually a gradual process, with signs and symptoms creeping up on you. Here are some things to look out for that may indicate you are on the road to burnout.

DISCONNECTION. A feeling of separateness from the people around you, like you're watching them from behind a window.

EMOTIONAL EXHAUSTION. Becoming cynical about everything and everyone. Little things become irrationally agitating. Small requests from loved ones start to really bother you.

CREATIVITY CRASH. At work, inability to think creatively leads to a declined work performance, which creates more stress and anxiety. At home, simple problems and obstacles mount up as you find yourself unable to think of a way through them.

INABILITY TO FEEL PLEASURE. You no longer are able to find pleasure in simple things. Pastimes and experiences that used to give you pleasure no longer do.

TIRED AND WIRED. You feel physically exhausted all the time and have no energy to do anything, yet you also struggle to sleep.

SELF-CARE SPIRAL. Your diet gets worse as you skip meals, snack late at night and begin comfort eating. You stop moving your body. You stay up later and later into the night, watching box sets and trash on TV as you try to unwind.

Please remember that many of these symptoms are not exclusive to burnout and can be seen in other conditions as well.

REDEFINING SUCCESS

Reliance on busyness to feel successful is the fastest track I know to emotional and physical sickness. It is crucial that we make a conscious effort to redefine for ourselves what "success" actually looks like. What should it look like to you? It is true that everyone has different lives with different pressures, so the answer to this will vary from person to person. But we also have a lot in common. Everyone has a basic need for inputs that aren't related to our work. We need time with family and friends, time to cook and eat properly, time to exercise, time to think, time to be in nature, time to pursue our hobbies and passions and time to rest. I believe a successful life is one that is broad rather than narrow, and the whole range of our basic human needs are fulfilled to at least a minimum degree.

What are the basic human needs? For me, they boil down to five things: work, family, friendship, health and passions. Each of these five needs are like separate fuel tanks. In a perfect life, each tank would always be full. But the reality is, it is very hard to achieve this. We only have so much time in our days, and it is very rare that anyone will be able to keep all their tanks filled up in the long term. Life has different seasons. In each season, we will find ourselves prioritizing certain fuel tanks. In our early twenties, for example, we may choose to prioritize our career at the expense of time with our partner and pursuing our hobbies and passions. In our thirties we may end up focusing more on our young children, if we have them, and consequently may end up not seeing our friends so much. In our forties, we may realize that we have neglected our friendships and some of our passions and start prioritizing them more.

As we go through life, and the demands that are made on us change, we will find ourselves making trade-offs as we focus on one or two tanks more than the others. This is fine. But it's also important to be conscious that we are making trade-offs, and aware that the more we neglect one tank, the less able we will be to thrive. Once we have this awareness, we can work to ensure that none of the tanks become completely empty – at least not for long. Sure, at times work will become so pressing that we will not have any time to spend pursuing our passions. But we should never allow ourselves to be in this state for long. Always keeping some fuel in each of the five tanks is a model of success that sets ourselves up for thriving, rather than burning out.

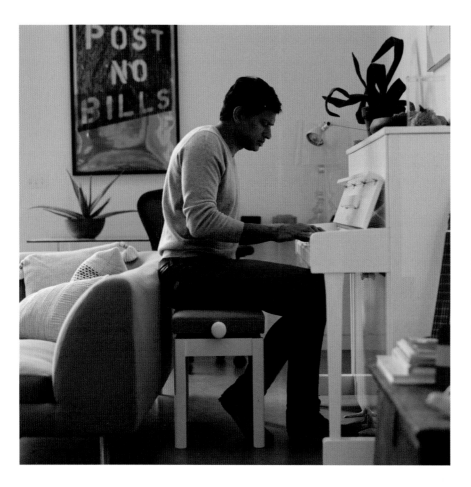
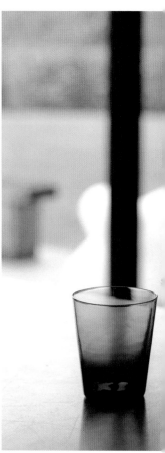
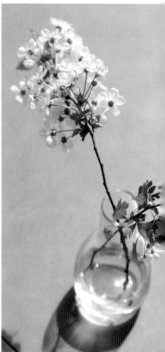

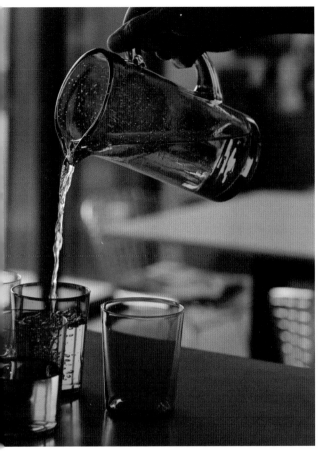

"A successful life
is one that is broad
rather than narrow."

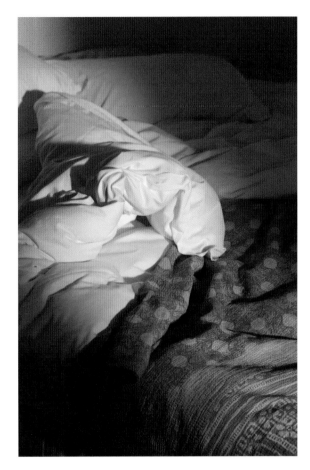

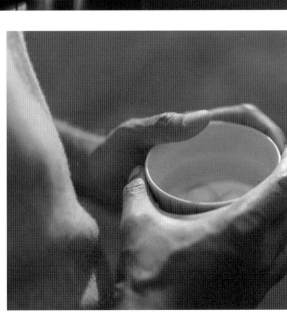

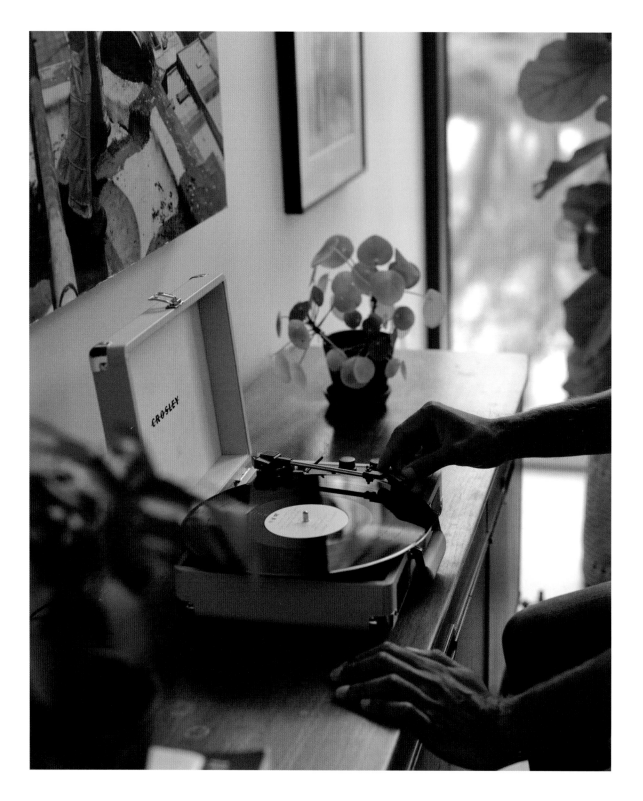

PROTECT YOUR REST

A huge part of keeping fuel in the health tank is protecting our rest. One of the most common upstream issues I have seen in the health of my patients is their inability to take their need for rest seriously. If we want to thrive, it's essential that we treat it as a non-negotiable. The best scientific research suggests that adults between the ages of eighteen and sixty should get around seven to eight hours of sleep a night, although this number will be highly individual. Professor Russell Foster from Oxford University recently shared on my podcast that working too much and depriving ourselves of sleep in the "peak years" of our forties significantly increases our risk of getting dementia later in life.

But it is also crucial that we understand what we actually mean by rest, in its fullest sense. We often think of rest in very narrow terms and equate it simply to having a nice sit down with a cup of tea or getting enough sleep. There's actually a lot more to it than this. Humans are active in three dimensions: they are physically active, mentally active and emotionally active. This means they must also seek rest in three dimensions: rest for the body, rest for the mind and rest for the heart.

BODY

The body requires physical rest, to restore it from the activities of the day. This could be sleep, light napping, relaxing on your sofa or Yoga Nidra, a relaxation practice that can be used in the day to rest and recuperate. There are many free Yoga Nidra videos on YouTube, if you wish to give it a go. Rest for our bodies does not really need much explanation because it's what we already naturally think of as rest.

MIND

The mind requires rest from the stresses and anxieties of the day. We're all surrounded by multiple demands on our attention, and each of these demands creates surges of neural and chemical activity in our systems.

When considering ways to mentally rest, a great rule of thumb is to think "analog" rather than digital. We're seeking a state of mental rest from overstimulation. Activities such as reading, listening to music, journaling, breathing practices, meditating or having a bath without scrolling your smartphone are perfect. Perhaps the ultimate form of rest and recovery for the mind is time in nature. On the evolutionary timescale, the built environment that most of us reside in is brand new. Nature is where we belong, and where the mind feels at home and unthreatened. When we are immersed in nature, we lower our cognitive load, and give our mind the space it needs to rest and recover. Just twenty minutes in nature lowers the stress hormone cortisol, helps us focus and be more present.

Perhaps surprisingly, the mind can also be rested by us losing ourselves in an active enjoyable pastime that takes our thoughts away from the stresses and strains of our lives. The organizational psychologist Dr. Sabine Sonnentag argues that what she calls "mastery" activities are a form of rest. These could be physical activities such as working out, cycling, tennis, or activities that mostly use your brain like learning a language, taking up a new hobby, playing a musical instrument, doing a crossword or playing board games. My wife Vidh had been suffering from brain fog for months, and found that it improved significantly when she took up the piano. She was getting enough sleep for her body. What cleared her problem up was getting enough rest for her mind.

HEART

The heart requires rest from our modern me-focused existence. Humans haven't evolved to be so separated from their human tribes and to be so relentlessly tuned into their own needs and ambitions. Rest for the heart involves doing something that connects you with other people, or something bigger than yourself. This could be volunteering, praying or studying sacred texts if you are religious or engaging in loving-kindness meditations that help you zoom out of your own life and think about spreading affection out towards others. You might also consider a book club, a game of pickup soccer, a drink in the pub or really anything that involves friendly face-to-face connection. Or, if that is not an option, it could be a phone call with one of your close friends or family. Even something as simple as sending someone a quick WhatsApp telling them how much they mean to you can be like a ginger-shot to the heart.

BODY	MIND	HEART
Sleeping	Reading	Volunteering
Napping	Listening to music	Praying
Relaxing on the sofa	Journaling	Studying sacred texts
Yoga Nidra	Meditating	Loving-kindness Meditation
	Breathing Practices	Connecting with others
	Time in nature	Taking part in team sports or community projects
	Taking a bath	Book clubs
	Learning a language	Phone call with a friend
	Doing a crossword	
	Taking up a new hobby	
	Playing a board game	
	Exercise	

GET UP TO SPEED WITH
THE ART OF SLOWING DOWN

Slowing down is an essential life skill we can all learn. It is also the secret of endurance. The very best endurance athletes in the world do 80 percent of their training at relatively slow paces, only going hard for 20 percent of the time. This is important to understand because endurance is something that we are all seeking.

I'm not suggesting that we all want to run marathons or cycle up mountains. Instead we want to endure in our own life as a partner, parent, colleague and friend, making sure we have the energy to be there for ourselves and others at the end of a long week, or indeed a long life. One of the simplest and most effective ways that I know of learning how to slow down is what I call the Push-Pause Method:

▶ What are the moments in your life when you feel pressured to rush? Might you be able to become more aware of them and consciously slow things down?

▶ What about when you get a message on your phone? What happens if you force yourself to wait before replying? What feelings come up for you? Do you feel anxious? Do you feel like you are failing somehow? Why is that? Are you able to pause your response and sit with that discomfort for five minutes? Then push it to ten minutes, and then more?

▶ What about when the person in front of you in the supermarket line is taking longer than you would like? Do you feel frustrated? Do you feel tension and stress building up inside you? By noticing these feeling, you can intentionally change your response. Perhaps, you could take a few deep breaths and remind yourself that those few extra seconds waiting really don't matter as much as you might think.

Over time, you will discover which situations in life lead to you rushing. And, by becoming aware of them, you are able to consciously slow things down if and when you are able to.

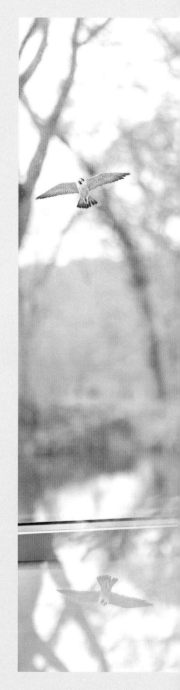

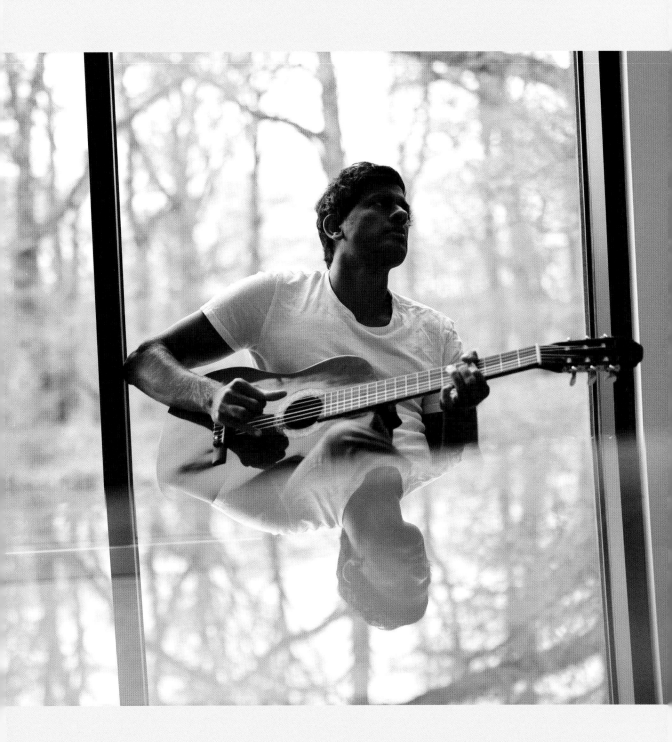

TAKE A SLOW DAY

When I was in high school, about a third of my classmates were Jewish. I often heard people talk about the Sabbath (known as "Shabbat") but I never really understood what it was truly about. A few years back, one of my friends, Suzy, invited me and my family to her house for Sunday lunch. While we were eating, she told me that, as a family, they stick to the Sabbath rigidly. It starts when it gets dark on Friday night and lasts until Saturday evening, and is a special day set aside for resting and relaxing with family. The word itself comes from the Hebrew *shavat*, which means "to rest."

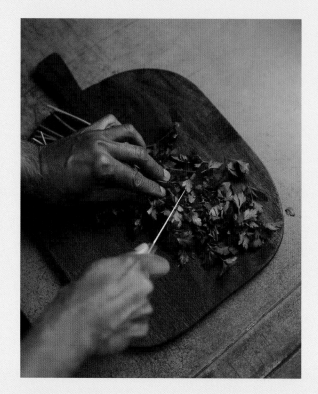

Because no work (including cooking) is permitted to be carried out on the Sabbath, all preparations need to be made the day before. Suzy told me that she prepares all of the family's food on Friday during the day and keeps it warm overnight in slow cookers. Over the Sabbath, the whole family will engage in restful activities like singing, lighting candles, playing games and enjoying special meals that can last for hours. They don't take phone calls or use any social media and are not permitted to do any "work." It is the ultimate experience of anti-busyness.

One of the things I noticed about Suzy's family was how close, friendly and joyful they were together. The atmosphere as we ate really captured the spirit that's so easy to lose, when family life becomes reduced to a series of chores and responsibilities that have to get done. As I sat and ate and absorbed it all, I felt I was in a truly wonderful place of listening, laughter and love. And, I have no doubt that the non-negotiable of their weekly Sabbath is one of the reasons why.

So much of the wisdom that is found in our religions is there because, over the span of time, it has been found to be beneficial. I believe that capturing the spirit of the Sabbath would be hugely beneficial for all of us, especially those of us with a reliance on busyness.

Once a week, I'd like you to think about taking a slow day. Ideally, everything that you do that day, would be carried out with the energy of slowness. Exactly what you do is up to you and will depend on the context of your life and your responsibilities, but here are some ideas to get you thinking:

▶ Walking slowly in nature – without your phone, if you are able to!

▶ Enjoying a leisurely breakfast without the pressure of finishing by a certain time.

▶ Driving 5 miles per hour under the speed limit – assuming it is safe to do so, of course! For some people, this will be extremely hard and demonstrate their constant reliance on busyness and speed.

▶ If you are going out for a drive, you could take a moment when you get inside your car to dust off the dashboard and give the seats a little clean, instead of just driving off as you might ordinarily do.

▶ Taking extra time to cook meals, with a real focus on the process rather than the outcome. Can you enjoy the time spent cooking? Perhaps you could listen to some music or a podcast you have not found time for during the week.

▶ Having a slow, relaxed lunch or dinner where you spend time eating, chatting, laughing and enjoying. The meal becomes something to savor rather than being something to quickly get done.

▶ Slow, mindful practices such as knitting or crocheting or painting.

▶ Working on a complex jigsaw.

To strengthen the power of your slow day, you could invite extended family or close friends to join in, which has the added benefit of nurturing relationships, something we will learn more about in Chapter 9.

If a weekly practice isn't possible, how about making it bi-weekly? If a full day is not possible, why not set aside the same three or four hours every Sunday afternoon or, perhaps, at a different time more suitable? Even just a few hours of "slow living" each week will help you feel calmer and more present. It will also make it much more likely that you are able to bring some of this "slow energy" into the rest of your week.

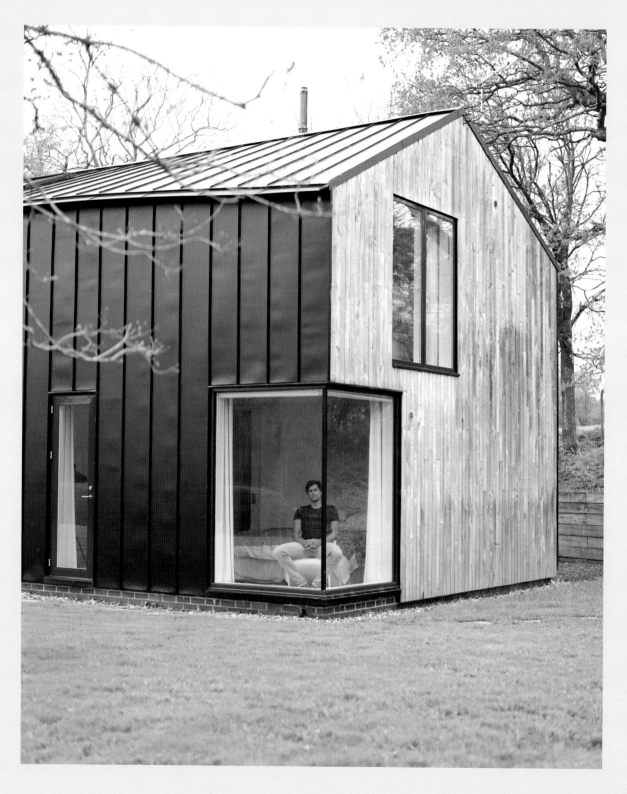

THE ANTI-BUSYNESS QUESTION

It's easy to fall into the trap of feeling that everything we have to do in life is of equal importance, when this is simply not the case. Some things are more important than others and many of us would benefit from developing the ability to ruthlessly prioritize. One of the best ways of doing this is to ask yourself the following question every single morning:

▶ What is the most important thing I have to do today?

This was one of the most popular questions in a short book I published last year, *The Three Question Journal*. Answering it daily has transformed my own life. Some days, I will write down something health-related, like going for a walk. Some days the most important thing will be to spend some uninterrupted time with my wife, or be fully present with my kids when they come home from school. On other days, it will be making sure I have the opportunity to walk to Mum's house and sit with her for an hour. And, on some days, it will absolutely be something related to work.

If you answer this question each morning and act on it, it is inconceivable that your life will not change. Too often, we think change is about the big things, like quitting a job or signing up for a Tough Mudder. But do not underestimate the importance of just focusing on the one most important thing in your life each day, every day, week after week and month after month. Small actions like these add up.

By answering this question each day, you bring into sharp focus what is truly important. Too many of us only attend to activities related to relationships, health and rest when everything else is done. The problem is "everything else" is never done, so we end up neglecting entire areas of our wellbeing. The ultimate cost of this can be deadly.

This is one of the best exercises to help you live a more mindful and purposeful life. Over time, you will find yourself intentionally focusing on what is truly important in your life. It will help you feel less busy and, as a consequence, you will feel calmer, happier and more in control.

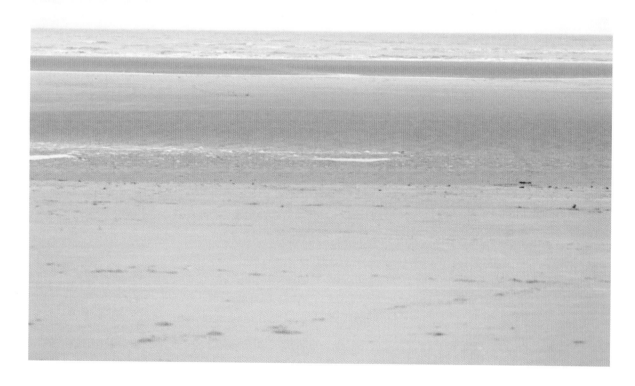

CONCLUSION

▶ Our culture equates being busy with being successful. This creates the toxic idea that, if we have space in our lives, we are failing. The reliance on busyness is widespread and incredibly harmful to our mental and physical health, and has caused an epidemic of burnout.

▶ To cut our reliance on busyness, we must have the courage to say no to things. We should embrace the fact that there will never be the time to do everything we want to, so we should prioritize the things that mean the most to us, and that we have to do. Every morning we should ask ourselves, "What is the most important thing I have to do today?"

▶ We should also intentionally redefine what "success" means to us. The five basic human needs are work, family, friendships, health and passions and it's helpful to think of each of these needs as tanks that need filling up. It's almost impossible in the modern world for anyone to keep all their tanks completely full. But a successful life is one in which all the tanks have at least some fuel in them most of the time.

▶ Prioritizing rest is also essential. Successful rest is about much more than sleep. Humans are active in three dimensions: physically, mentally and emotionally. This means they must also seek rest in three dimensions: rest for the body, rest for the mind and rest for the heart. If possible, we should also introduce a weekly "slow day" into our schedule.

9. GIVE MORE THAN YOU GET

The gift of reliance

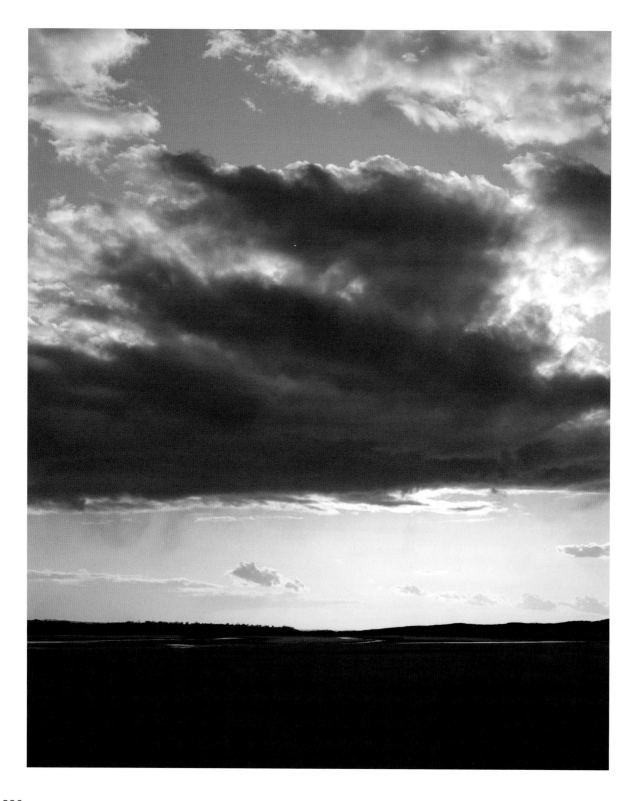

I'll never forget the call. It was February 8, 1998, I was twenty years old and studying medicine at the University of Edinburgh. It was shortly after 11 p.m. and I was chilling in my flat when the phone rang. It was Mum. She told me that my father had been suddenly taken into hospital. He was in intensive care and the doctors weren't sure if he was going to survive the night.

"I think you should come home now," she said.

"Sure," I told her. "I'll try."

I put the phone down and slumped against the wall, bewildered and in a state of shock. I was 240 miles away. How on earth would I get back to Cheshire? I didn't own a car and there were no trains or coaches at that time of night. I was standing in the hallway when my roommate, Steve, walked in through the front door. He had been working late in the library as he had an exam the following day, which counted towards his end of year assessment. I told him about the phone call and he helped me call around. It soon became clear that there was going to be no easy way for me to get myself home that night.

"Why don't I drive you?" he said.

"No, you can't," I replied. "You'll be late and exhausted for your exam."

"It's fine, mate. I'll get you home, put my head down for two hours and then drive back up to Edinburgh."

"I can't ask you to do that, Steve. Thanks, mate, but it's too much."

He threw his keys at me.

"Let me just grab a few things. Meet you in the car in five."

I recently thought about that weekend again for the first time in years. It was 9:45 on a Friday night and I heard a beep alerting me that I'd received a text. It had been a long day, and I had somehow forgotten to turn my phone off, which is what I typically would do about an hour or so before bed. I reached to get it and was about to shut it down when I saw the message was from an old friend of mine, whom I hadn't spoken to in ages. "Hi, mate, I'm in a really bad way," it said. "I really need to talk to you urgently. Can you call me now? Please."

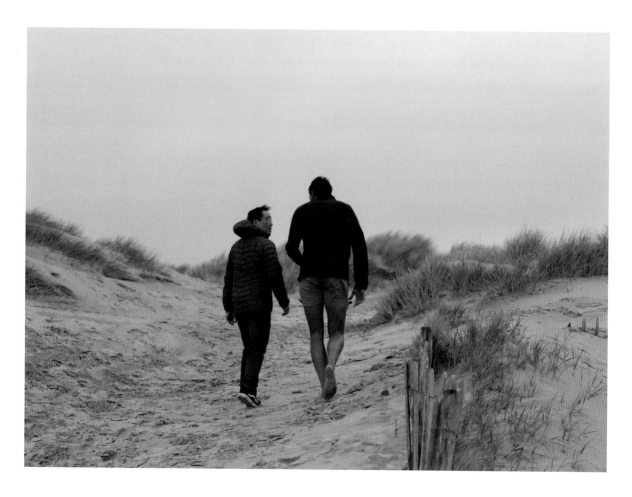

For me to get back to someone at that time of night was exceedingly rare. I would always absolutely prioritize my sleep. But I remembered how amazing Steve had been for me, years ago, and it was obvious that Matteo really needed me now. So, I went downstairs, found a quiet place, and spent an hour on the phone with him, talking through the problems he was having in his marriage.

Both of these incidents involved reliance. Two decades ago, I had relied on Steve to take me to my dad when I needed him. The other night Matteo relied on me, in an admittedly much more modest way, in his moment of need. This is reliance done properly. Every single one of us will fall down, at multiple points during our lives, whether due to relationship and family issues or work problems or in episodes of illness, grief and despair. We'll need to be able to reach out to people around us and be vulnerable and supported. When others do this for us, it's a gift. But when we allow ourselves to be relied upon, we are also given a gift. The day after I spoke with Matteo, I was definitely tired and not as productive at work due to my late night. But I had zero regrets. He had reminded me that I am a good friend who is always there for the people I love, no matter what. And for that I was deeply grateful.

OVERDOSING ON FREEDOM

All the way through this book, I have made a point of stressing repeatedly that our goal should never be zero reliance. I'm aware that the danger with this minimally reliant philosophy is that once we start cutting the invisible reliances that are holding us back, we will start thriving and loving it – and then take it too far.

As strange as it might sound, it is certainly possible to achieve too much freedom. For that we have to thank millions of years of human evolution. Our species has been designed by nature to function optimally in the form of highly cooperative groups. This means that we just don't have the power to be self-sufficient. We can't survive and thrive on our own. We are supposed to receive help from others in order to live well. It's how we're built. But it also means that we're supposed to be the source of help for the people around us. The gift of reliance runs in both directions. When we give and when we receive, we always benefit.

"The gift of reliance runs in both directions."

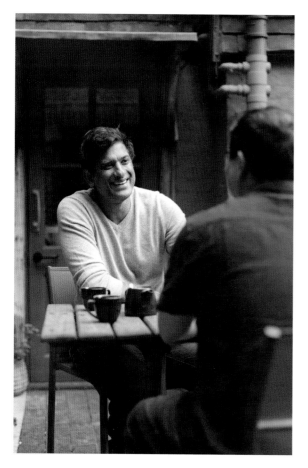

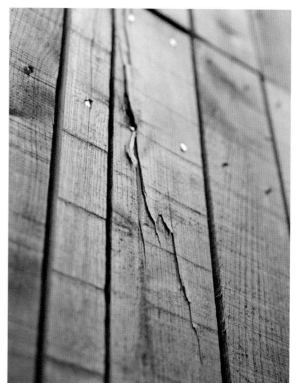

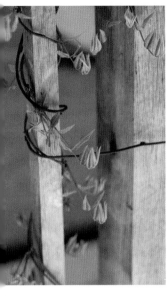

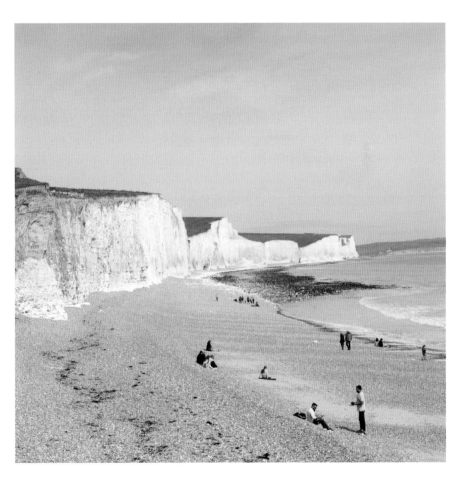

That's why it is so important that we don't take things too far. There's a real risk that pursuing minimal reliance to an extreme could leave us isolated and being perceived as a little standoffish, selfish and egotistical. Some people become so attached to the idea of being independent that they find it difficult to reach out and ask for help when they are struggling, sometimes with tragic and devastating consequences. We should never forget that no matter who we are, we'll always exist within a community of other people. Even the individuals we hold up as heroes only achieved what they did with the help of huge numbers of helpers. So many of us fall into the trap of thinking Steve Jobs invented the iPhone by himself, that Elon Musk is solely responsible for inventing the self-landing space rocket and that Taylor Swift alone is responsible for all the songs she sings and the concerts and videos she performs in. After all, it's these men and women who receive almost all the credit. But their achievements also belong to the huge communities of professional supporting individuals, many of whom are just as talented and hard-working as the heroes who stand in the spotlight.

The crucial thing to know about our communities is that they are there to help and support us – but they need to be nourished in the form of the help and support that we provide. This state of mutual reliance is a core part of being human, and we turn our back on it at our peril. There is overwhelming evidence that having strong social connections has massive downstream effects on our physical health. One major study has found that people over seventy years old with strong social connections were 22 percent less likely to die over a period of ten years. Another study, of around 3,000 women with breast cancer, found that those with at least ten friends were four times more likely to survive their disease than those with no close friends. The evidence is inarguable. We'll suffer terribly if we sever all our ties completely. The more connections we have, the more likely we are to thrive.

"The more connections we have, the more likely we are to thrive."

FINDING MINIMAL

When Steve offered to drive me down to Manchester, he did so because he truly cared about me. But I wonder if he would still have been so ready and willing to stop his revision and risk being too tired to do his exam if I had asked him to? Would he have done it if this wasn't the first time I'd needed an emergency lift, but the fifth? And what about when Matteo needed help from me? Would I have taken the hit on my wellbeing the next day if he'd had a habit of always asking me for help? The honest truth? Probably not.

Just as having zero reliance can leave you isolated, living your life in a state of maximal reliance will also leave you vulnerable. Because we evolved for millions of years as members of highly cooperative groups, humans have finely tuned subconscious detectors for people who exploit the benefits of our communities. When someone behaves in a way that's greedy for resources like food or cash, you can be sure the people around them will notice. But this is also true when they're greedy for their community's emotional resources. When anyone over-relies on the good folks around them for love, attention and empathetic concern, you can be sure people will realize, and realize very quickly.

So what is this ideal state of minimal reliance that we're pursuing? It's simple: that we give more to others than we receive. To achieve this state, we need to take control of the things that we are overly reliant on and work on changing our mindsets so that we no longer need them as much. This is a matter of building psychological and physical resilience in all the ways outlined in this book. Soon, we will find that we have become strong enough that we can choose whether we want to treat ourself to a sugary snack or a lazy Netflix session or a doomscroll on social media. But we will be free of the need to do any of these things. With this inner and outer strength, we will also find that we will be calling on the help of others with much less frequency. This means that when we are genuinely in need, we can be sure that people will rush to our side to be of help.

When we're truly thriving, there is never any shame in allowing ourselves to be caught on the days that we fall. We are a gift to other people. But we're not fully human if we don't allow other people to be a gift to us too.

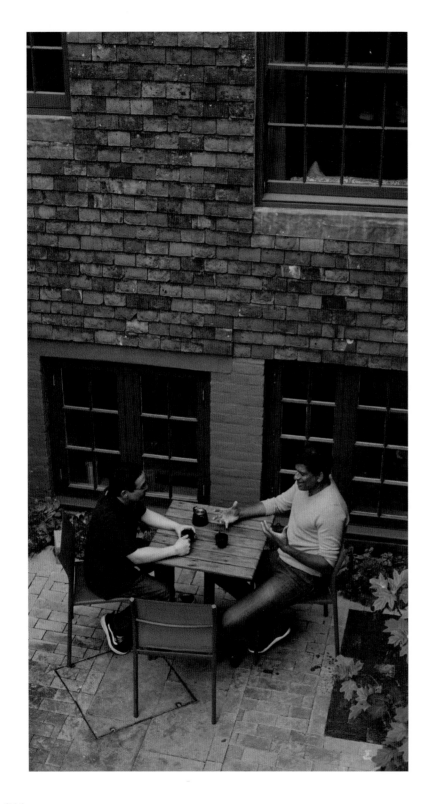

THE FOUR SOCIAL CIRCLES

Over the last ten thousand years, it seems that human life has transformed completely. We were once members of nomadic tribes that roamed the forests and savannas. Then we invented farming and settled down in packages of land we called our own, giving rise to a world of kings, queens and conquering emperors. Now we largely live in an era of government, markets and advanced technology. But if you peel back the layers of all this astonishing progress and focus on the fundamentals of how we live our lives, and what we need to thrive, almost nothing has changed. We are, as we have always been, incredibly groupish. We are designed to thrive when we are plugged into networks of other humans. When we become unplugged from our networks, our emotional health and our physical health begin to crack and crumble. We become sick and depressed.

This need for social reliance also exists in those animals who are relatively close to us on the evolutionary tree. In one scientific study, rhesus monkeys were removed from their troop and then had biopsies taken from their lymph glands. The tests showed that these isolated monkeys had significantly increased their levels of inflammation, which – as we've discovered elsewhere – makes us humans vulnerable to cancer, heart disease, diabetes, arthritis, bowel disorders and a host of other conditions. This had happened because the monkeys' brains took their isolation as a signal: they were in danger. Just like humans, rhesus monkeys cannot survive on their own. And, just like humans, their brains are continually listening to the signals that are given out by the world around them that tell them if they're thriving – or if they're not.

These signals are critical to thriving. Humans exist in social tribes on four different levels and, ideally, we need regular positive signals from each level to feel good. The widest level is community. Our community is our tribe. Twenty thousand years ago it would've been the band we belonged to that roamed about hunting, gathering and setting up camp in the bush. Today our community is the people we see as we move about our lives: our neighbors, the workers in the shops, restaurants and coffee shops we see regularly, fellow commuters at bus stops, platforms and carriages. At the next level down are our friends. Whether we've known them since we were children, or since our children met their children, our friends are those that we can rely on, and that we know intimately. At the next level is family, both nuclear and extended. And at the heart of it all is our partner, that one person we have chosen, above all others, to rely on and to offer our own reliance.

SQUARING THE CIRCLES

We can think of these levels as social circles. In order to truly thrive, each circle will ideally be complete, meaning we'll be successfully connected to our community, friends, family and partner. It's important to note, though, that depending on our individual circumstances, this might seem an impossibly high bar to reach. If one of our circles is broken in a serious way, it's important to identify this and compensate where possible. For instance, if we're not lucky enough to have a close family, we can actively compensate by strengthening our bonds with our partner or friends. In the same way, if we don't have a long-term partner (either through choice or circumstance), we can compensate in the friends or family circles. One of my patients, who struggled for years with his family and friendship circles, started volunteering at the listening helpline Samaritans. He found that the new relationships he developed with his fellow Samaritans, and the intense conversations he had with his callers, provided all the social signals he had been lacking. Because of this, his volunteering work made him happier than he had ever been.

We should also acknowledge and accept that life is nonlinear. As we explored in Chapter 6, we can't rely on the belief that nothing in our lives will ever go wrong. The ups and downs we naturally experience mean that we will go through periods in which some of the circles will become broken for a time. Recently, I was on stage with Professor Rose Anne Kenny, an expert in the aging process, and she was describing the experience of loneliness. As she was talking about how common social isolation was, and how much we need regular interaction with friends, it suddenly hit me. I became quite emotional. I realized that yes, I am pretty lonely right now. This is because my life is filled up with work, family and all the time that's necessary to look after my mother. What's taken the hit, in all this, is my friendship circle. Mum's declining health has definitely impacted my ability to fully thrive, for the moment. But I understand that this is a choice I have made, it's a choice I don't regret and it's not forever. This is how life is. While it's important we are conscious of the health of each social circle, it's equally important that we don't create an over-reliance on them all being complete at all times.

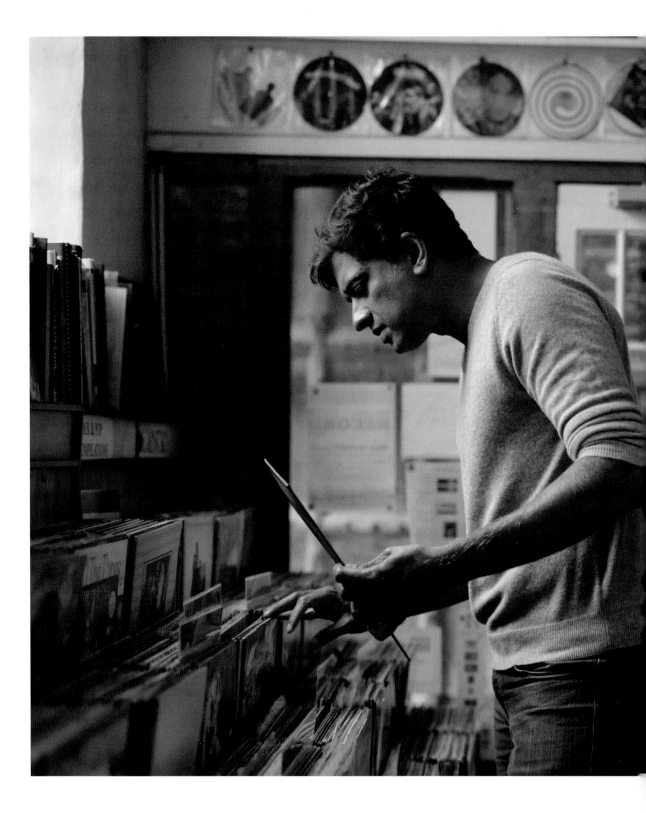

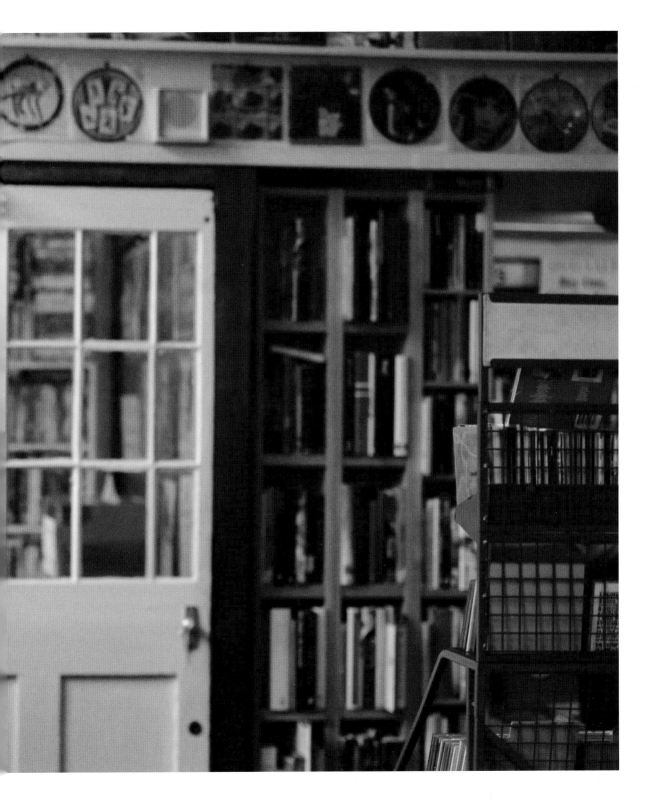

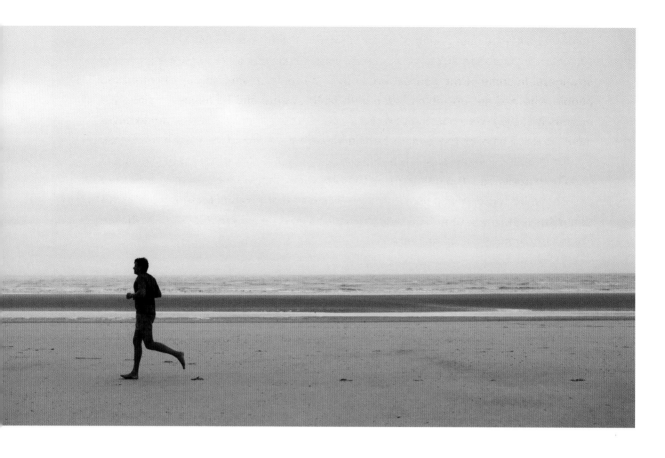

RELIANCE ON COMMUNITY

One of the greatest lessons I've ever learned about the power of community was when I ran the London Marathon in 2021. The honest truth is, I shouldn't have taken part in the event that year. I was injured and in a huge amount of pain, to the extent that, between miles ten and twenty-six, I could barely lift my right leg. I had to literally drag myself through the final half of the race. I didn't burst through the finish line covered in smiles and glory but with a grimace and a feeling of "thank God that's over." As a physical experience, it was hellish. But, in another way, the experience was truly wonderful. What I witnessed as I hobbled through the streets of London was the most incredible example of community reliance.

When we spend time online, or watching the news, we're continually given a very powerful signal that the world is hopelessly divided by politics, race, gender and class. Everyone hates each other and the dream of us all coming together as one human family is almost a kind of childish joke. But that is not what I saw for those six hours in October 2021. What I saw was thousands of strangers supporting strangers. In some of the poorest areas that the route travels through, I witnessed people who had set up tables laden with fruit, sweets and homemade cakes and muffins that they were passing to runners, people they didn't know and would never meet again. Some of the people behind those tables would very likely have had opposing political views to some of the runners and had very different backgrounds and life experiences. It didn't matter. The Marathon showed me how able we are to rise above our petty divisions. Of course, I realize that humans often fall out about things they find important. But our conflicts don't define us. What makes us who we are is our capacity for community.

And I really felt it that day. From the bottom of my heart, I know I would never have gotten over the finish line if it hadn't been for those strangers lining the streets and cheering me on. They gave me a gift. And I'm pretty sure the runners gave them a gift in return. The joy on their faces as they called shouts of encouragement and handed out drinks and delicious cakes said it all. Despite my physical pain, I had an awesome experience. I truly witnessed the beauty of humans when we are at our best.

COLLECTIVE EFFERVESCENCE

Readers of my previous book, *Happy Mind, Happy Life*, will already know how beneficial I believe it can be for us to talk to strangers. The nods of hello at passers-by in the park and the snatches of small talk shared with people behind counters in shops and cafes can change the tone of our day. Scientific researchers argue that this kind of social connection is so important that it amounts to a kind of social vitamin, or "vitamin S," that we should take daily. It helps us thrive because it's a regular signal that tells our brains that we are members of a supportive tribe: that the strangers we share our lives with are not to be feared; instead they are good people that we can rely on when in need.

But it's not only in streets, parks, cafes and shops that we have the chance to take vitamin S. We can also have powerful experiences of communal joy, which researchers sometimes call "Collective Effervescence," when we go to concerts, films, plays, clubs or even parties. Collective effervescence is a primal tribal phenomenon that seems to trigger something deep in our humanity. Whenever I think about it, I'm reminded of the famous Oasis concert at Knebworth in 1996 (a staggering 2 percent of the entire UK population tried to get tickets for the gig). When the event took place, the police reported hardly any problems with the crowd. Those who were lucky enough to go and sing along to "Champagne Supernova" with 125,000 other people, would have had an experience of collective effervescence so intense they would probably never forget it.

But you don't have to attend once-in-a-lifetime concerts to experience the joy of community. You could attend yoga classes, join a choir or go to your local comedy club. In this post-pandemic era, making the extra effort to physically be with other people has never been more important. Yes, it's convenient and easy to talk to people via Zoom, or watch videos of events on the YouTube app on our phones. But when we deprive ourselves of the positive signals that come with true human presence, we make it impossible for ourselves to thrive. One telling scientific study showed that people laugh thirty times as often when they're with other people compared to when they're alone. This tells me how crucial it is that we have regular experiences of ourselves as successful members of the great human family. And we can only do that by getting up off the sofa and out of our front doors.

NO MAN IS AN ISLAND

I know from the patients I have seen at my practice that social isolation is a problem that hits middle-aged men especially hard. I suspect this is part of the reason that middle-aged men are more likely to commit suicide than any other group. In earlier generations men would often have socialized in local pubs. A negative consequence of the otherwise positive decline in alcohol use is that we now have far fewer places where men can just hang out and chat and feel connected to a friendship group.

As I know from my own experience, middle age is often a time when our lives become completely filled with work and family responsibilities. We can easily lose touch with childhood mates and, especially in the working-from-home era, struggle to make true friends of the people we work with. For whatever reason, women seem to be able to make social connections far more easily than men. In my local park, I've long noticed how common it is to see women strolling in pairs and chatting happily, while men often walk alone.

Psychologists characterize male friendships as "shoulder-to-shoulder" and female friendships as "face-to-face." In other words, men tend to bond by doing active things together, while women more typically bond by sharing their inner thoughts and feelings. This profound understanding has led to an international "Men's Shed" movement. Started in Australia, it seeks to create new places where men can meet and bond while learning new things together, whether it's lawnmower repairs or furniture restoration. I love the idea of this, and strongly encourage my male readers to try to take the maintenance of their friendship circles as seriously as they do their work. And if your partner is a man who has a broken friendship circle, I'd urge you to do whatever you can to encourage them to get shoulder-to-shoulder with other men.

But whatever your gender, it's important for all of us that we regularly spend time laughing and sharing who we are with a circle of people that we trust, care for and have a shared history with. The reliance on friendship is a reliance on people who accept us warts and all, who will be there for us when we need them, and who will remind us of our value when we show up for them.

RELIANCE ON FAMILY

A few years ago, my wife's mother came to stay with us for five weeks. I know that some people would be concerned about how this might go but I was actively looking forward to it and feeling relaxed. The experience was fantastic and eye-opening. Having just one extra adult around, helping out with cooking, cleaning and the kids, was a revelation. The entire dynamic in the household changed. The kids seemed happier and Vidh and I became closer as well. We seemed to have more time to chat with each other, were able to go out for walks together and our marriage became revitalized almost overnight.

Those weeks made me think about how unnatural the nuclear family is. The modern world has brought us many good things, but often at the cost of our emotional health. As we have explored in previous chapters, our money- and status-driven culture drives up levels of perfectionism and fools us into thinking that busyness equals success. But the prevalence of the nuclear family is yet another shift that we have not evolved to deal with. In ancient human tribes, grandparents were always on hand to help with parenting – as were uncles, aunts and friendly neighbors. My short time living with my mother-in-law gave our family time for things that weren't about the basic daily necessities of eating, getting ready for school, homework, tidying and everything else that fills our schedules. It wasn't only each other that Vidh and I had more time for, we were also more available for our two children. If Vidh's mum was cooking one evening, it meant we could play together with our kids, or kick a ball around in the backyard. These simple moments of pleasure and play were wonderful to experience. But they were also bittersweet. I got a sense of what life could be like if, collectively, we could just carve out a bit more time in our lives for our families.

The social circle of family is one that depends, more than any other, on the giving and receiving of reliance. Our children absolutely rely on us to be there for them and give them what they need, while we desperately want them to grow up as we wish them to and learn to thrive. Just as with the social circles of community and friends, these reliances are gifts that we both give and receive. The danger with family is that we forget to make space for activities that aren't simply about the completion of responsibilities and chores.

I don't believe a family can truly thrive if its members rarely laugh and play together. I was given a powerful lesson in this only recently. Over the past few years, my relationship with my brother has become dominated by responsibility, as we negotiate the care of my mother. He would often come to my house to talk about the situation, or organize something for the next day; on occasion, the mood between us would become serious and somewhat tense. Noticing this, I started to suggest we play a couple of games of snooker when he arrived. Just ten minutes of play would transform the tone of the conversations we would then sit down to have. It sent us both a signal that reminded us that we are brothers, that we love each other, and that even though the situation isn't great, there is still a lot more to our relationship than our mum's care.

RELIANCE ON OUR PARTNER

If we are lucky enough (and have consciously made the choice!) to have a partner, this will likely be our most important relationship. Committed couples willingly fuse their lives together. Mutual reliance is the very definition of what long-term monogamy is. It's the gift we give each other every day. But our relationship with

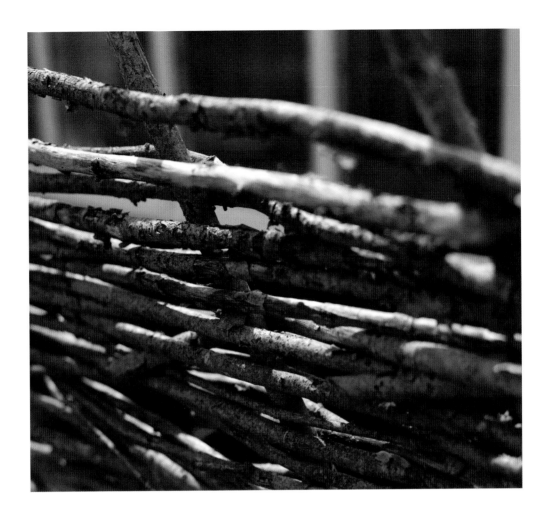

our partner is vulnerable to a huge amount of wear and tear. If there is a problem in any of our other social circles – our community, friends or wider family – we all too often take it out on the person closest to us. This is one of the reasons achieving minimal reliance is so important. The more self-reliant and immune to stress, strain and temptation we become, the more we will be able to give to our life partner.

We will also make space for the reliances that brought us together in the first place. When you met your partner, they probably made you feel good about yourself physically, made you laugh and made you feel special, wanted and heard. These are such hugely valuable reliances, but they can be fragile, especially when we hit middle age. A relationship that thrives is one that nurtures these tender reliances and places a high value on keeping them strong.

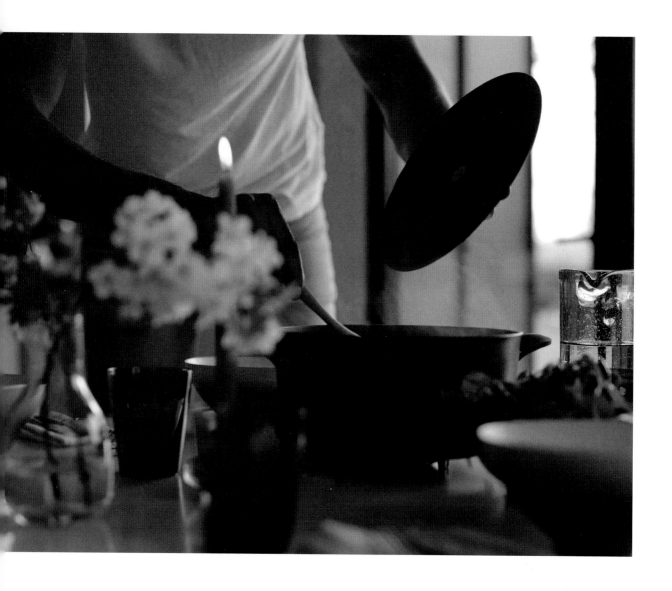

I was recently inspired when I read about Marc Randolph, the co-founder of Netflix, who always makes a point of making Tuesday night date-nights with his wife. "I resolved a long time ago to not be one of those entrepreneurs on their seventh start-up and their seventh wife," he wrote. Even when he was working flat out at the growing company, he explained, "rain or shine, I left at exactly 5 p.m. and spent the evening with my best friend. We would go to a movie, have dinner, or just go window-shopping downtown together. If you had something to say to me on Tuesday afternoon at 4:55, you had better say it on the way to the parking lot. If there was a crisis, we are going to wrap it up by 5:00."

Throughout these pages I've already covered plenty of advice that has helped me in my relationship with my wife Vidh. Whether it's never imagining you can read the mind of your partner or being clear about communicating your boundaries (see Chapter 3), there are so many ways in which pursuing a philosophy of minimal reliance can strengthen your closest relationship. But the gift of reliance is also critical to it. In making his Tuesday date-nights a non-negotiable, Marc Randolph was ensuring that he and his wife continued to rely on the things that are so easy to forget in a long-term relationship. He was creating the conditions for his most important relationship to thrive.

THE GIFT OF OTHER PEOPLE

Some of the worst places in the world are prisons. These are buildings specifically designed for the punishment of human beings. They are as close as we get to hell on earth. And what are the worst places inside any prison? The segregation units. Prisoners that break the rules are thrown into solitary confinement, which has been shown to increase their psychological distress, shorten their lives and, sometimes, cause a permanent change to their brains and personalities. This is the closest we have, in the West, to a legal form of torture. The worst thing that the state is allowed to do to a citizen is to separate them from other humans.

This is the danger of pursuing zero reliance. We cut ourselves off from the great human family and accidentally build a prison of isolation for ourselves to exist in. But going too far the other way is also dangerous. Maximal reliance means we demand too much of our social circles. We become needy, weak and exhausting. We wear them out. The sweet spot is minimal reliance. We should strive to become strong enough that we can give more than we take. But we should never forget to be human enough to enjoy what others give us.

ASSESS YOUR SOCIAL CIRCLES

When you have space, think about the current state of your own four social circles: community, friends, family and partner.

For each one of them, ask yourself, how they are currently being nourished. Score them from zero to three

0 — This circle is not being nourished at all.

1 — You are doing the bare minimum.

2 — You are doing a pretty good job but could do with a little more focus.

3 — You are nourishing this circle well.

Then, write down one action you can take this month that will help further strengthen each social circle. This could be making sure you have some intentional time alone with your partner each week, a phone call with your parents or an in-person catch-up with your siblings or friends.

If you struggle to nurture ties with your community, why not consider which hobbies or activities you enjoy and join a local class? This is such an effective way of building up local networks with people who have similar interests to you.

When you're doing this exercise, please remember to be kind to yourself. This is not about beating yourself up, it's simply about making an honest and accurate assessment of your social health. Remember, for many of us, it can be challenging to keep all of the circles fully nourished at all times. But by thinking about our reliance networks consciously, we can spot areas that are in need of repair, and begin to mindfully fix them.

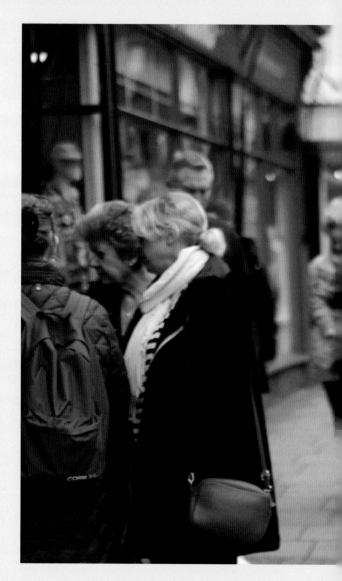

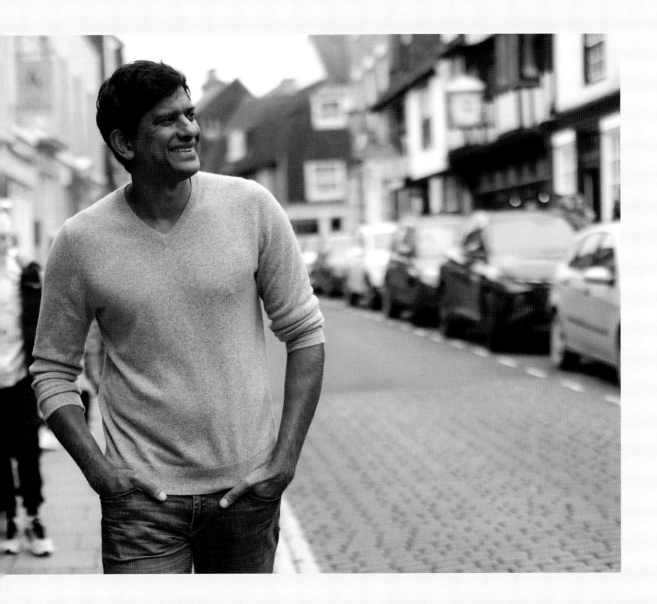

CONCLUSION

▶ It's critically important that we don't take the pursuit of Minimal Reliance too far. Humans are a social species, and a certain amount of reliance is not only advisable – it is essential. A huge amount of research shows that social connection is critical for good health. Our goal should be to always give to others more than we expect in return.

▶ All humans have potential access to four social circles – community, friends, family and partner. From time to time, we may end up going through periods of discomfort in each of these four circles, but we should always pursue a life in which each of them is complete. If any of them are incomplete, either through choice or life circumstance, we can compensate by strengthening our bonds in the others.

▶ Other people are a gift, and we should be able to rely on them when necessary. When we achieve Minimal Reliance, and give more than we take, we will become a wonderful gift to the people in our lives.

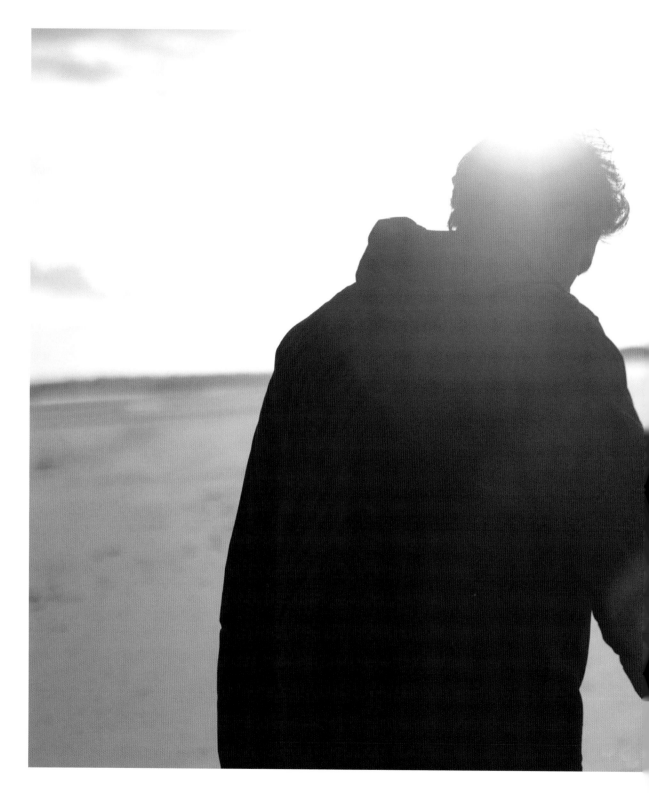

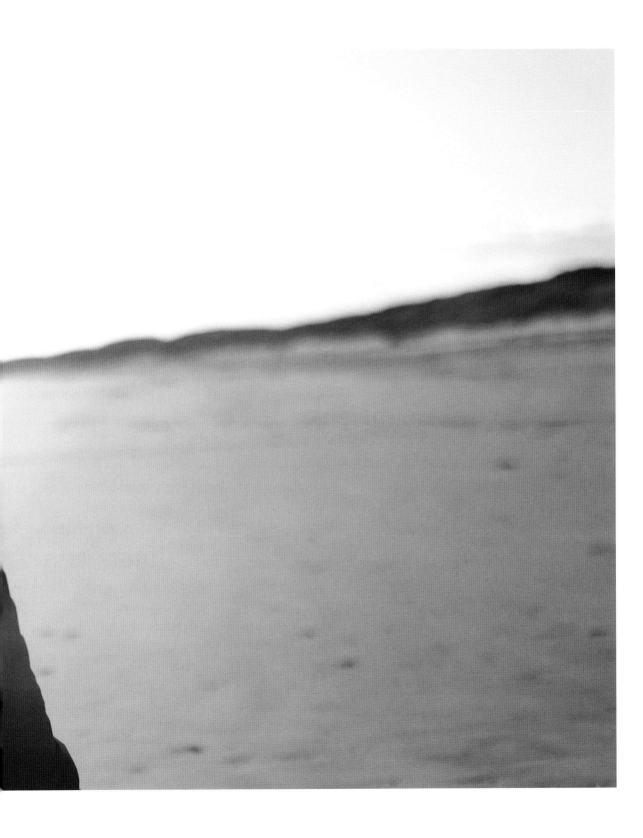

TIME TO THRIVE

Throughout my career I have been fascinated by the relatively small upstream changes we can make to our lifestyles that will have huge downstream benefits for our overall lives. The philosophy of Minimal Reliance is the result of more than two decades of thought, practice and observation. It is incredibly powerful because as soon as we become less dependent on our invisible reliances, we immediately start to transform our health and happiness.

It is no exaggeration to say that learning to see the world through the lens of our invisible reliances has changed my own life. It has certainly changed the lives of many of my patients. It is my experience of putting this concept into practice that has convinced me of the huge potential it has for all of us. It is how I know that what you hold in your hands is much more than just a book. Minimal Reliance is a way of life that is simple to understand yet based on cutting-edge research. It is one of the most powerful ideas I know for anyone who wants to truly transform their emotional and physical health.

As enthusiastic as you might feel right now, my advice would be to start small and spend some time finding a daily practice that helps you get to know yourself better, as detailed in Chapter 1. Learning to listen to yourself, and becoming a world expert in you, is an essential first step to achieving minimal reliance. It's also worth remembering that all of us are dependent on different things in order to thrive, so I would encourage you to reflect on each of the 9 chapters and think about which ones moved you emotionally and resonated the most. It might be worth revisiting those chapters and spending some time focusing on the ideas and practices within them. You might also want to experiment with trying practices from just one chapter, embedding them in your life in modest ways that grow slowly but steadily, week after week. Then start adding in practices from additional chapters. Very quickly you will find that you are becoming stronger and healthier in surprising ways.

▶ You will grow in confidence.

▶ You will experience less stress.

▶ You will become kinder and less reactive.

▶ Your physical health will improve.

▶ Your mental health will improve.

▶ You will feel happier.

▶ Your friends, family and colleagues will begin to like and admire you more.

▶ You will become the kind of person who gives more, who takes less and who others want to be around.

▶ You will feel more in control of yourself, and of the world around you.

To put it another way, you will have learned how to make change that lasts.

REFERENCES AND FURTHER READING

CHAPTER 1. TRUST YOURSELF: RELIANCE ON EXPERTS

https://www.theguardian.com/science/2021/aug/15/the-hidden-sense-shaping
-your-wellbeing-interoception
https://www.thelancet.com/journals/eclinm/article/PIIS2589-5370(21)00322-9
/fulltext
https://pubmed.ncbi.nlm.nih.gov/30928884/
https://pubmed.ncbi.nlm.nih.gov/32172039/
https://mbl.stanford.edu/sites/g/files/sbiybj26571/files/media/file/zahrt-apple
-watch-2023.pdf

CHAPTER 2. GIVE UP YOUR HEROES: RELIANCE ON PERFECTION

https://www.apa.org/pubs/journals/releases/bul-bul0000138.pdf

CHAPTER 3. BE YOURSELF: RELIANCE ON BEING LIKED

Gabor Maté, with Daniel Maté, The Myth of Normal (Vermilion, 2024)
https://www.ncbi.nlm.nih.gov/pmc/articles/PMC1823975/?page=2
https://pubmed.ncbi.nlm.nih.gov/9603702/#:~:text=Results%3A%20
Increases%20in%20the%20number,stressful%20events%20one%20week%20
later

CHAPTER 4. EMBRACE DISCOMFORT: RELIANCE ON COMFORT

https://www.bmj.com/company/newsroom/physical-inactivity-is-responsible-for-
up-to-8-of-non-communicable-diseases-and-deaths-worldwide/
https://www.sciencedirect.com/science/article/pii/S2667137921000072
https://www.npr.org/sections/health-shots/2013/11/20/246316731/kids-are-
less-fit-today-than-you-were-back-then
https://www.science.org/doi/10.1126/science.aap8731
https://www.ncbi.nlm.nih.gov/pmc/articles/PMC5025014/
https://www.healthline.com/nutrition/10-health-benefits-of-intermittent-fasting

CHAPTER 5. TAKE LESS OFFENSE: RELIANCE ON BEING RIGHT

https://www.health.harvard.edu/staying-healthy/understanding-acute-and-
chronic-inflammation
https://www.ncbi.nlm.nih.gov/pmc/articles/PMC3839356
Adam Grant, *Think Again* (W.H. Allen, 2023)

CHAPTER 6. EXPECT ADVERSITY: RELIANCE ON THINGS NEVER GOING WRONG

https://www.thegrocer.co.uk/supply-chain/shrinkage-costing-uk-retailers-almost-11bn-a-year/594726.article
https://www.bmj.com/content/362/bmj.k4016
https://greatergood.berkeley.edu/images/uploads/Frias-DeathGratitude.pdf
https://www.sciencedaily.com/releases/2012/04/120419102516.htm
Bronnie Ware, *The Top Five Regrets of the Dying* (Hay House, 2019)

CHAPTER 7. LET GO AND MOVE ON: RELIANCE ON THE PAST

https://aacrjournals.org/cancerres/article/79/19/5113/638250/Posttraumatic-Stress-Disorder-Is-Associated-With
https://pubmed.ncbi.nlm.nih.gov/2047503/
Bessel van der Kolk, *The Body Keeps the Score* (Penguin, 2015)

CHAPTER 8. BUSYNESS IS NOT SUCCESS: RELIANCE ON FEELING IMPORTANT

Will Storr, *The Status Game* (William Collins, 2022)
https://hrreview.co.uk/hr-news/wellbeing-news/88-have-experienced-burnout-in-the-last-2-years/145535
https://www.cdc.gov/sleep/about_sleep/how_much_sleep.html

CHAPTER 9. GIVE MORE THAN YOU GET: THE GIFT OF RELIANCE

https://pubmed.ncbi.nlm.nih.gov/15965141/
https://pubmed.ncbi.nlm.nih.gov/16505430/
https://pubmed.ncbi.nlm.nih.gov/25870391/
https://journals.sagepub.com/doi/abs/10.1111/j.0963-7214.2004.00311.x
https://www.samaritans.org/about-samaritans/research-policy/middle-aged-men-suicide/
https://www.irishtimes.com/life-and-style/health-family/loneliness-the-hidden-unspoken-issue-affecting-middle-aged-men-1.4042590
https://en.wikipedia.org/wiki/Men%27s_shed
https://www.moneycontrol.com/europe/?url=https://www.moneycontrol.com/news/trends/why-netflix-co-founder-marc-randolph-leaves-work-at-5-pm-on-tuesdays-9810261.html
https://www.ncbi.nlm.nih.gov/pmc/articles/PMC7546459/#:~:text=Such%20studies%20have%20found%20that,aggression%20%5B14–16%5D
https://www.prisonpolicy.org/blog/2020/12/08/solitary_symposium/
Robert Waldinger and Marc Schulz, *The Good Life: Lessons from the World's Longest Study on Happiness* (Rider, 2023)

INDEX

ACKNOWLEDGMENTS

Writing books is one of the most rewarding pursuits in life, yet one of the most challenging, as well. To put down your ideas in a way that is accurate, engaging and easy to understand is a skill I will spend my lifetime trying to get better at. Although it is my name that is printed on the cover, the writing of this book was absolutely not a solo pursuit. It was only possible because of the incredible support networks that I am blessed to have around me.

A huge, heart-felt thanks to my mum and dad, who have devoted their lives to giving me and my brother the best start in life that they could. I am eternally grateful.

To my wife, Vidhaata, thank you for believing in me, loving me and supporting me in everything that I do. Thanks also for the wonderful edit suggestions that have immeasurably enhanced this book.

To my wonderful children, Jainam and Anoushka, you both mean the world to me and are the inspiration behind all that I do.

Thanks also to my brother, Barun, for always being there for me, and to Chetana and Dinesh, the best in-laws anyone could hope to have in their lives.

Beyond my immediate family, there are so many wonderful people in my life who continually provide me with love and support. In contrast to my previous books, I have decided to not mention every single person by name in this one – you all know who you are.

A special thanks also to the whole team at Penguin Life, Will Francis, Will Storr and Rich Gilligan.

I would also like to acknowledge the contribution of every single person I have ever interacted with, both offline and online. I have long held the belief that we can learn something from everyone and that has certainly been my experience to date. Whether it has been a positive interaction or not, I can assure you that I have learned something about myself from each and every one.

Lastly, I would like to thank you for choosing to spend some of your precious time with the words I have chosen to share. I truly hope that they have resonated and inspired you to think about your life differently, and I hope that they continue to do so for many years to come.

ABOUT THE AUTHOR

Dr. Rangan Chatterjee is one of the most influential medical doctors in the UK with over two decades of clinical experience and his mission is to help 100 million people around the world live better lives. He is Professor of Health Communication and Education at Chester University, host of one of the world's most popular health podcasts, *Feel Better, Live More*, and the author of five *Sunday Times* bestsellers. He regularly appears on BBC television and national radio and his TED talk, "How To Make Disease Disappear," has almost 6 million views.